The *Vital* Truth

Accessing the possibilities of unlimited health

"*The Vital Truth* reveals the essence of true natural healing.
It explains how Chiropractic care, along with the amazing inborn intelligence of
the human body, can bring about
the greatest vitality and a most renewed well-being."

Dr. John F. Demartini
Best selling author
Count Your Blessings - The Healing Power of Gratitude and Love

Dr Sarah Farrant

First Published 2007

2nd Reprint 2009

Published by Bountiful Pty Ltd

The ideas, information, suggestions and procedures in this book are purely those of the author and are not intended as a substitute for consulting with your health care provider. The author does not accept responsibility for any action, claim, adverse effects or consequences resulting from the use of any idea, information, suggestions or procedures contained in this book.

The names of individuals whose stories are used in this book have been altered to protect the privacy of the individuals concerned.

Cover design by Ben Mathieson, Bees Knees Designs.

Layout and design by Toni Esser, tesser book and print design

Edited by Jo Hopping, editonline.

Printed by Vervante

ISBN 978-0-9803185-0-0

This book is dedicated to
individuals all over the world
who would love to have
health and vitality in their
life through the power
of increased internal
communication.

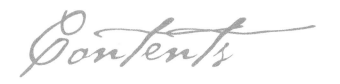

Contents

Acknowledgements

When writing this book I had a feeling it was never going to end. There was so much I wanted to share, teach and inspire people with about vitalism and health, where it comes from, how to gain it, and how to keep it. Inspirational in my quest to complete this book has been my husband. Unwavering in his strength and support, he has stepped in to give me the space I have requested in order to complete the journey. Our two boys, Anam and Rui, and our newborn little girl, Anais, have been patient as Mum has set about interacting with them whilst sending a fax, printing a page, writing an article or researching material! Thank you all for your love, encouragement and optimism. I am truly grateful.

To "Little One". The lessons and teachings you gave to me enabled my life to be changed. I gained so much from the experience I shared with you. I am grateful for the opportunity you gave to me to be your mother.

There have also been friends and other family members who have shared in my journey. To my parents, John and Sue, and to my sister Lisa, thank you for the life journey we have shared thus far. Those experiences have so aptly framed a part of this book. I feel blessed to be sharing this lifetime with you all.

To Kim and Sunny, I give heartfelt thanks of gratitude. When the times got tough your words of encouragement enabled me to soldier on.

Thanks must also go to D.D. Palmer and B.J. Palmer for their insight and genius in founding and developing the Chiropractic profession. They have impacted my life and the lives of millions around the globe.

Thanks to Dr. Lea Piche and Dr. Alison Asher for reading and providing pre-print input. Your feedback has been invaluable.

Thank you to my editor, Jo Hopping, for believing in my message. You have encouraged me to look at new ways of expressing principles and above all, to keep going!

The invitation

The time has come to embrace a different perspective on health. A new understanding of health is developing: where it comes from, what it is, how to get it and importantly, how to keep it. Individuals are daring to ask questions and to do life differently.

The old habits of thinking about health are giving way and the emergence of the new paradigm has the power of an art, a science and a philosophy to back it up.

It was after the birth of our second son, Rui, that I was given a vision to share vitalistic philosophy and how it relates to health at a global level. I went to have a lie down one afternoon after I had put our two boys to sleep. Before sleeping I asked what I was meant to do with my life now I was contemplating staying at home to focus on raising our children, rather than return to practice full time or even part time. Upon waking, I was quite stunned and overwhelmed at the vision that had been shared with me. Tears filled my eyes as I began to write the message down. This is what I was told:

"To share vitalistic philosophy with the world and how it relates to health, for the purpose of changing the health consciousness of individuals, families, communities, cities, states, nations and the world; to inspire a desire in others to do their life differently; to ask different questions."

I had gone to sleep that day asking a different question and I was prepared to hear the answer, as overwhelming as it might have seemed at the time. In sharing this health perspective with you I have chosen to share my own life experiences and the factual experiences of others who have crossed my path in my professional career. The book is written in sections to help you digest the material presented. It is a pick up/put down type of book, or one that can be read from front to back. At the end of each chapter is "The Vital Truth", a summary to remind you of the important points, and "The Vital Questions" for you to consider as you take the journey through the book. The aim is to provide you with a sound understanding of what truly constitutes health and where it comes from. In doing so, my wish is to provide you with a balanced perspective. Balance is important, not only in health, but in every area of our lives.

This book is based on three basic principles:

1.   Health exists on a continuum

2.   The power that made the body heals the body

3.   Nature needs no help, just no interference

Join me as we journey through this new interpretation of health. It is my wish to share this knowledge with the world and it starts with you. The impact will be global, and sharing it with individuals, families and communities can affect cities, states, nations and the globe. So as we journey, I ask you to put down any preconceived ideas you may have regarding health, what it is, and where it comes from, clear the mind, and be open to seeing new ways.

It is my vision that you will find the balance in your own life and in your own health, and in so doing share this knowledge with friends, family, partners, husbands, wives and children over dinner, in the park, at school, or at any other social event. With your help the impact can be vast. Together we can lead a new way of thinking.

Thank you for allowing me into your home and your heart. Enjoy discovering "The Vital Truth".

DR. SARAH FARRANT

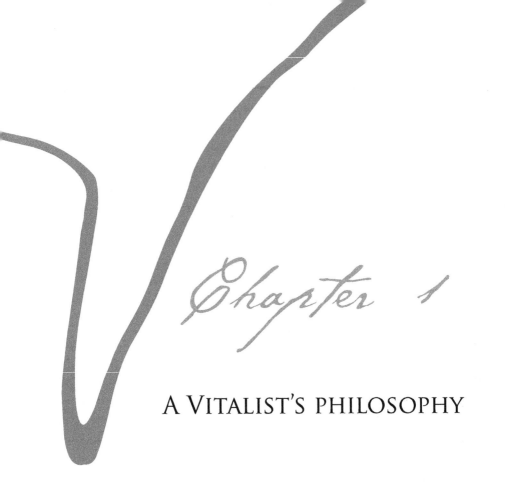

Chapter 1

A Vitalist's philosophy

"If you continue to think as you always thought;
you will continue to get what you have always got."

ANON

The mechanist and the vitalist have been arguing with each other for well over 2500 years about what actually constitutes health and disease and what signs and symptoms represent. This argumentative view of health and medical history was first postulated in writing by Harris L. Coulter, Ph.D., a great medical historian. In *Divided Legacy* (Volumes 1-4)[1] Coulter traces the vitalist/mechanist division as it permeated history. The following is what I have found to be the major differences between the two schools of thought.

Vitalism respects the structure and function of living things while at the same time recognizing that there is an "innate intelligence" that designed and keeps the systems working as they should.

Our bodies are intricately designed. If left to its own devices, the innate intelligence that so perfectly assembled your body is easily capable of healing your body during your physical lifetime. Yet we have been taught to place our trust in other people to such an extent that we've lost our courage and our trust to let our innate intelligence do what it does best: to balance and to heal.

It's imperative to understand that there are things which can affect our body's ability to communicate with itself and so bring complete healing. These are known as thoughts (emotional), trauma (physical) and toxins (chemical), or the "3Ts". It's also necessary to understand the differences between a mechanistic and a vitalistic philosophy if we are to realign our thinking and see real change.

The mechanistic theory (sometimes known as atomist, rationalist or allopathic theory) views the smallest components of the physical body's structure as building blocks. These blocks are understood to make up the whole. From the smallest component of ourselves we see vibrations, then subatomic particles, then atoms and molecules which build tissues; which in turn form organelles, organs, and systems. This view, however, leaves no room for an "innate intelligence", looking only at problems in isolation rather than in the complete interconnected form. The mechanistic approach maintains that the body is powerless to perform self-maintenance and healing. This assumption places a higher value on the educated mind than on a body that actually made itself. It also assumes a "fix it" mentality and has the user take on a passive participant role.

Newton established "universal laws" that helped us understand the movements of the planets and tides, and his Mathematical Principles of Natural Philosophy was the standard by which science came to be measured. Yet his findings didn't seem enough to explain the kinds of life that seemed more than an assembly of parts. Ordered growth and development seems best understood when an innate intelligence is incorporated.

Until 1932 the mechanistic view of health was widely accepted. Then something astounding happened. Ernst Rutherford split the atom and discovered that "matter" was comprised mostly of "space". This seemingly empty space was actually a large amount of energy unable to be seen with the naked eye. Einstein realized energy played a critical role in keeping the atom together and in the process he brought vitalistic philosophy back into the limelight.

Since the 1950s the mechanistic philosophy has wavered. Doctors who were once respected were now being questioned. The Baby Boomers questioned authority in the '60s, challenging everything from scientific thinking to health choices. Mass media made spreading new values an easy process and today people are making informed choices about their philosophy, their values and their health care.

> VITALISTS BELIEVE THAT "SOMETHING" – AN ESSENTIAL ENERGY – IS RESPONSIBLE FOR ORGANIZING THE HUMAN BODY TO KEEP IT FUNCTIONAL.

A vitalist senses that it is not enough to understand the "building blocks". Vitalists believe that "something" – an essential energy – is responsible for organizing the human body to keep it functional. This "intelligence", this life force, this energy, is the difference between a corpse and a living body.

Yet vitalism isn't new. Hippocrates was a vitalist. Born Hippocrates of Cos in 460BC, his name became synonymous with Greek philosophy and he wrote the "Oath of Medical Ethics" which is still in use by medical physicians today.

Hippocrates held that the body must be viewed as a whole rather than a series of parts. He believed in the natural healing process of rest, good diet, fresh air and cleanliness. Ironically, what Hippocrates taught and where the mechanist understanding of health and disease finds itself today appear to be two different viewpoints.

The wisdom of the body is far greater than anything we can conceive. Let me give you an example of how the innate intelligence affects the entire system of the body at once: Joan came into the practice a few years ago. She had been everywhere with her shoulder complaint and surgery was the next option for her. She wanted to see somebody else about it before she made that decision. I asked Joan why she thought she had this sore shoulder and why it started in the first place. Like many who think in a mechanistic paradigm she said "I don't know. I was just reaching up into the cupboard and then I couldn't move it." I asked her how long she'd had it for and she replied that it had been a few months. So my next question to Joan was "How has this sore shoulder served you over the past few months?" She wasn't too sure about my question, so I asked her again. She looked quite perplexed at the thought of there being a benefit to her having a sore shoulder. As we went along she started to see the benefits. She'd had a break from cooking meals, she was driven around, her husband had taken time off from work to help more around the house, and the children became more independent. At the beginning of the consultation, Joan was only seeing the pain without the pleasure. Joan's sore shoulder was giving her benefits in her life, I am certain of that. She could see the only way this was going to change was by changing the way she thought about it. I also explained to Joan how the body is interconnected. I explained her sore shoulder could be coming from the hips, neck, or cranium, which then results in postural changes and altered states of health expression.

The postural changes Joan adopted in order to decrease the discomfort she was experiencing had an effect on the organs, too. The nerves exiting a particular nerve root port were under compromise which further meant a system or systems could have been affected. So, Joan had symptomatic expression in the shoulder area which brought her in for a consultation. We recognized that the expression could have been coming from anywhere (thoughts/emotional, trauma/physical or toxins/chemical – 3Ts) and that there were benefits and drawbacks to the situation and creation of the discomfort. We also surmised that this altered state of health expression might also have had an impact on her various organs and ultimately, systems.

When the body has everything in balance, it is better able to express health to its fullest potential.

The mechanistic approach to health care assumes that everybody is the same on the inside. We are as different on the inside as we are on the outside! I remember at the age of ten driving in the car with my mother to see "the family" medical doctor who just happened to be my uncle. It was a rainy day and I stared out the window as we drove, pondering what he was going to do, tell me and give me. My mum, because of the paradigm she was living in, was probably driving there thinking this visit would help and provide some relief. Relief to whom? I had a sore throat and I remember saying to Mum, "He's not going to do anything; I'll just get another tablet to take." When I went in to see the "Doctor" he looked down my throat, noticed the tonsils were inflamed and sure enough gave me Amoxil, one of the more common antibiotics. From that day forth I rarely mentioned to my parents details of any type of health challenge I faced. I knew innately that seeing something in the body in isolation wasn't going to help, but instead would probably hinder my ability to build an immune response.

I share this story because when we look at the back of prescription packets we tend to see a plethora of side effects. This variety comes from the variance in people. People react in different ways as a result of the 3Ts - thoughts, trauma and toxins (or emotional, physical and chemical), their structure and function at the time, their values and their perceptions of life. We truly are as different on the inside as we are on the outside.

If we know that we are so unique on the inside, why would we put something into our bodies that we know could possibly harm us?

> PEOPLE REACT IN DIFFERENT WAYS AS A RESULT OF THE 3TS – THOUGHTS, TRAUMA AND TOXINS (OR EMOTIONAL, PHYSICAL AND CHEMICAL)...

Vitalism brings a different approach to health care. The innate intelligence of the body which created it really does have the ability to heal it. What happens when we cut our finger? The body heals it. A whole chain of events takes place in just the right sequence, in just the right amounts and at just the right time in order for the platelet coagulation to take place at the site of the cut.

My husband and I are constantly telling our children that their bodies heal themselves. Our bodies are so intricate that man hasn't yet been able to replicate a single cell. We need to let go of our search for a "quick fix" for our health and not imagine that it has, in fact, been lost. We never lose health because our bodies are constantly searching and reorganizing themselves in order to continually express health. In fact, we never lose anything in life. Whatever we perceive to be missing is always there – we just have to look. It's usually in a form that we have not yet recognized.

Health is always inside of us. What can change, however, is its expression.

Within the vitalistic model there is greater incentive to be the observer in one's ability to express health. This "way of life" philosophy enables us to check in with ourselves, to awaken ourselves to our imbalances and to search each day for the answers we need for our health and make choices accordingly.

A different level of responsibility goes with this way of thinking. We are responsible (or should we say "response-able") for our health. People who are comfortable with this philosophy will recognize the internal wisdom of the body and its ability to heal itself. With this knowledge, people tend to make healthier choices.

Mechanism

Vitalism

Mechanism	Vitalism
There is no intelligence in the universe; chaos dominates and existence happens by chance.	All living things are sustained by a vital force. Everything is maintained in existence in a perfect order.
When bodies are compromised in some way, health is added to it from an invasive, outside-in approach to gaining health: e.g. surgery, nutrition, exercise, food, medicine.	Health is gained from the internal workings of the body, coordinated by the nervous system. People have everything they need to heal themselves, provided there is no interference. People are awakened to their imbalances by a lack of "ease" in the body
The person becomes the passive participant in their search for health; an external person is in control of their health and well being. Responses are based on a fear of pain.	The person is the active participant in their search for health. People respond best to trust in their ability to maintain their health. Vitalism supports living without fear.
The body is equal to the sum of its parts — believing that the smallest component of matter is the atom which has no intelligence or consciousness.	The body is greater than the sum of its parts. This model recognizes that an energy exists, and from that energy matter and life emerge.
Disease comes from the outside and must be gotten rid of. Bacteria and viruses cause disease and must be eradicated.	Bacteria and viruses are an essential part of our ecosystem. Care is taken not to interfere with the natural functioning of the person in order to protect other functions.
Sacrifice for the good of the whole e.g. vaccinate all children knowing that some will die and some will be irreversibly damaged.	Childhood "diseases" are normal developmental steps for a healthy child.

The 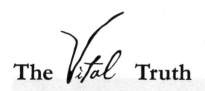 Truth

- The essence of life is housed in a vitalistic philosophy.

- Vitalism recognizes there is a (g)rand, (o)rganized (d)esign to the flow of life.

- The body is a temple for growth and health expression.

- Nothing is ever lost or gained.

- The body gives us signs and symptoms for the benefit of finding out more about ourselves and the imbalances with which we are living.

The *Vital* Questions

- Write about a time in your life where you have incorporated the vitalistic philosophy.

- In what way have you found your body to heal itself other than a cut finger?

- Write about a situation where you, a friend or family member have healed their body and ultimately changed their life through this vitalistic understanding of health.

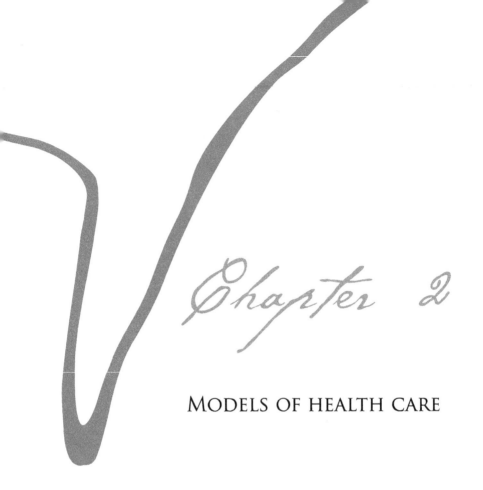

MODELS OF HEALTH CARE

"Hidden away in the inner nature of the real man is the law of his life and some day he will discover it and consciously make use of it. He will heal himself, make himself happy and prosperous and will live in an entirely different world. For he will have discovered that life is from within and not from without."

RALPH WALDO EMERSON

There are three models of health care available today: the medical paradigm, the complementary and alternative medicine (CAM) paradigm, and the *real* alternative!

The medical/mechanistic paradigm is one we all know too well. It is an "outside-in" approach to apparently regaining some form of "health". In correspondence to The British Medical Journal,[2] Ron Law noted that preventable medical errors in hospitals are responsible for 11% of all deaths in Australia and New Zealand. Adding deaths from properly researched, properly registered, properly prescribed and properly used drugs to the preventable deaths results in a figure that covers 19% of all deaths. Law then noted this is almost 1 out of every 5 deaths. This should astound you.

The National Health and Medical Research Council (run by the Australian Government) states that we spend 8-10% of the Gross National Product on health care. Yet 60% of Australians were sick within the last 2 weeks, 60% of Australians take drugs for a chronic health problem, 50% of adolescents are taking painkillers and 40% of 15 year olds suffer some kind of chronic disease.[3]

Do you think the country is in a health care crisis? Do you think the government needs to seriously consider restructuring how health is interpreted? Why are we perpetuating the myth that health is found in a pill? People and governments are perpetuating a sickness industry where conglomerates and bureaucracies have the ability to dictate who gets what, when and where. Who are the ones who prosper? The pharmaceutical companies. This allopathic model demonstrates a disease-centered focus. A person miraculously "gets" a disease and of course something from outside the body heals it, takes it away. You are seen as "unlucky" to have had disease strike you and are viewed as disadvantaged. The "doctor", under this model, is seen to be almighty and powerful with the patient as the passive participant. It's interesting that the allopathic model is concerned with treating the disease and not the cause. Medicine truly is disease care. Medicine has its place in trauma care, emergency care.

The complementary and alternative medicine (CAM) paradigm is very similar to the allopathic model. The key difference is that they are doing the same thing but with herbs, oils, candles, massage. I'm not saying that people are unable to help themselves by using these methods, however I am saying that this is still working and providing care in a treatment paradigm, which is perpetuating the myth of disease being bad. When people have a massage the massage therapist will undoubtedly ask if there are any areas of complaint. The massage therapist, for example, works on the shoulders a little more, or perhaps the lower back, if the person receiving lives in this model and tells the therapist where the area of complaint is. Whatever the symptom, the person in the CAM paradigm is ultimately treating something. For instance it doesn't matter where I am around the world, e.g. Bellagio, Las Vegas or a remote island in Fiji — when I receive a massage the approach seems to be the same. The masseur/masseuse asks me if there any areas of complaint which need attention.

The ALTERNATE paradigm is where vitalism truly sits. A profession which takes a stance on vitalism and embraces its understanding is the chiropractic profession. It is not a substitute for medicine — far from it. Some medical doctors would like to think it is, as they set about implementing spinal adjustments to people without the proper training. Chiropractors are the only ones educated and trained thoroughly enough in the neurology of the body to deliver adjustments to people. The profession, under the guidance of this vitalistic philosophy looks for the cause of the symptomatic expression, rather than treating the disease. The chiropractic profession puts emphasis on the occurrence of an internal disruption, an imbalanced perspective and/or neurological compromise when people have changes or departures from their once-ideal expression of health.

CHIROPRACTIC IS A PHILOSOPHY, A SCIENCE, AND AN ART WHICH CONCERNS ITSELF WITH THE RELATIONSHIP BETWEEN STRUCTURE AND FUNCTION.

Chiropractic is a philosophy, a science, and an art which concerns itself with the relationship between structure and function. When these are in balance, we see an evolution take place alongside a restoration in health and a preserving of life. Chiropractic truly is health care.

It has been my observation over the years that there are three levels of health care in Chiropractic today. First is initial intensive care which is designed to assist the body and mind to help itself in reducing symptomatic expression and therefore find balance and stabilization internally. It is important to note here that although symptoms may be reduced or eliminated, this does not mean a return to health.

In a symptomatic state there is approximately a 30% loss of function within the body. Just because we don't have the symptoms any more doesn't mean we are necessarily fully functional once again. Now, we don't just wake up with the dis-eased state, do we? No — it happens over a period of time. Imagine you have been asked to a party by some friends, however the host's place is in a suburb where you have never been before. You get in the car and wonder to yourself "how am I going to get there?" Invariably, you look up the road map. In not knowing where you are going, you stop and start as you look at the map. Upon arrival you partake in the social festivities and find that during the return journey you seem to get home far more quickly than it took to travel to the party. I have noticed this scenario in my own life time and time again.

Health is no different. It takes time to decrease the health expression in the body because the body ultimately wants you to be in a state of balanced health expression at all times. It can take years before the educated mind gets any signs and symptoms from the innate (inborn) intelligence, suggesting it raise its awareness to the imbalances in life. However when we begin the journey to unravel the messages being received by the educated mind from the innate intelligence, the journey seems so much faster – and it is. We become awakened to the understanding that there is divine order in the innate intelligence within and we gain new insights into our lives. The question is: is it necessary to wait until we get signs and symptoms before we become awakened, or is there something we can be doing on a regular basis that helps us to see and gain the balance in life?

The next level of health care is based on health restoration. *Dorland's Pocket Medical Dictionary* and the World Health Organization define health as "a state of optimum physical, mental and social wellbeing and not necessarily the absence of disease or infirmities." There is no mention in this health definition about having "pain" or "no pain" or "signs" and "symptoms". Health is truly about reaching optimum, not average, but optimum levels of expression in all areas of life (see Chapter five). It is more than prevention or maintenance, which simply imply having reached a desired level at which maintenance now takes place.

It is important to remember here that we have deconstructive and constructive forces acting on us all the time. Let's have a closer look at this before we move on, as this is an important point to grasp. We have within us deconstructive forces and constructive forces occurring constantly. We also have deconstructive forces within the environment and constructive forces internally helping to destroy and build us. We are the builders and destroyers of our own bodies. Right at this moment while you are reading, there is apoptosis occurring (cell death) as well as cell development and growth, at the exact same time. The purpose of this level of health care is to aid the body in correcting the long standing CAUSE of the perceived loss of health. It is about peeling back the layers. Think of the body as an onion where you are working to get to the centre point, the balance point, and the true essence of who you are in all areas of life. This level of care works at a cellular level, where the cells are able to rejuvenate and the innate intelligence of the body is once again on its way to health, and ultimately, wellness expression.

The third level is wellness care. It is based on function and adaptation. Wellness is a journey of self-discovery in not only the physical realm, but also in the spiritual, mental, vocational, financial, familial and social realms. It is an "active participant" process of increasing our knowledge base, which enables us to make wiser choices which ultimately take us to a more balanced existence. By this definition, wellness care is about ongoing care designed to optimize our life expression. Our possibilities for health are endless and our health is only limited by our minds. We are all beings of infinite possibilities, beings of perfection. Anything is possible.

When I do introductory health talks in the practice and in the community at large, I find it fascinating to note the responses I get when people are asked: What is health? Most reply that health means not having to take medication, feeling good, not having symptoms and being fit and eating the right foods. Not many people can answer what health truly is and where it comes from.

NOT MANY PEOPLE CAN ANSWER WHAT HEALTH TRULY IS AND WHERE IT COMES FROM.

In 2002 my husband and I traveled around Florida giving radio interviews and talks at various Universities. Whilst I was at one particular University I decided to find the medical school and ask some of the students what they thought health was and where it came from. I came across a young African-American man in his mid to late 20s and asked if he wouldn't mind sitting and having a chat with me for awhile. He was kind enough to oblige. I knew he didn't know what type of conversation we were going to have. I was direct, as I like to be, and I asked him why he had chosen medicine as his vocation. He shared with me that he wanted to provide for his family more than his parents provided for him. So my next question was: what is health? He responded that it is having no pain, having no symptoms. When I shared with him the definition of health I like to use, the one from *Dorland's Pocket Medical Dictionary* which states health is "optimum physical, mental and social wellbeing and not necessarily the absence of disease or infirmity", he was stunned. He had no idea about this health definition. In fact he shared that, to date, the professors at the university had not yet defined what health was. He was in tears when we finished our conversation hours later and thanked me for the encounter. He sent me an email some months later thanking me and sharing that he had just been to the medical school admissions office and had withdrawn from the course in the hope of finding something more supportive of his newly-acknowledged values and understanding of health.

The key to health is FUNCTION. The purpose of the nerve system — central nerve system (brain and spinal cord) and peripheral nerve system (everything else) — is to control and coordinate the function of all the cells, tissues, organs and systems in the body, and to relate and adapt the body to its internal and external environment. This is an important point. Everybody's external environment is different. Our environment, what it is that we choose to see, is based on our own perception of reality. This is why the internal balance of an individual is proportional to their function and adaptability to the external life. This balance does not come from the digestion of medications, but from the art of balancing the nerve system. Medications are designed on the theory that everybody is built the same way. We are not.

So when the chiropractic profession mentions the key to health is FUNCTION, it suggests that if our nervous system is working in a coordinated manner, thus allowing the parts of our bodies to function 100% of the time all the time, then we are more likely to reach optimum states of balance and health expression. We would then truly have a state of optimum physical, mental and social wellbeing which would then provide us with new opportunities to do our lives differently.

When we operate at this level of awareness, contemplation and balance, there are limitless possibilities as to what the body and mind can be, do and have on a daily basis and well into the future.

The 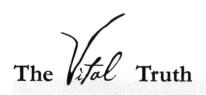 Truth

- There are three models of health care available to the consumer.
- The first is a treatment paradigm with medications.
- The second is a treatment paradigm with alternative remedies.
- The third is a true ALTERNATE model where you must make a paradigm shift in your understanding of health and where it comes from to adopt this understanding as a way of life.
- The chiropractic paradigm says an optimally functioning nerve system is able to adapt to life externally and internally, and in so doing, raise the awareness of individuals to do their life differently, to ask different questions.
- The quality of your life is based on the quality of the questions you ask.

The Vital Questions

- Which model of health care are you attracted to?
- In what level of care do you reside (initial care, health restoration, or wellness care?
- In what ways can you be or become an active participant in your own health care?
- Are you ready to ask the questions, or rather, are you ready to hear the answers?
- What level of health care do you want for yourself, your family and your friends?
- What level of responsibility are you ready to have toward your health?

Chapter 3

INNATE INTELLIGENCE

"Natural forces within us are the true healers of disease."

HIPPOCRATES

There are many professions out there that claim to be in the business of health. There aren't many professions out there, however, that recognize the presence of an internal wisdom within the body — an innate intelligence, if you will, that runs the body. This innate intelligence is responsible for giving the body life; it is what separates life from death. Innate intelligence is in all organic matter, from the complexities of the human being to the single-celled organism. It is complete in us all from pre-conception through to death. It does not discriminate. It is no different in a young child than in a ninety-nine year old woman; it doesn't change with our level of education or the school we attended or whether we are a genius or mentally challenged. All living things have this innate intelligence. It is the one great thing that treats us as equals. It gives organization to the smallest functioning parts of the body, which then gives rise to the cells. It then gives organization to the cells to form tissues and to the tissues to form organs and then to the organs to form the systems of the body. The only thing that separates a living body from a corpse is this presence and expression of innate intelligence.

This term "innate intelligence" was coined by D.D. Palmer who founded the chiropractic profession well over a century ago and it is what B.J. Palmer referred to as the Law of Life. Innate intelligence, he said, was the internal understanding of the body that knows what to do every time, all the time, all day and night for the rest of our physical lifetime. In recognizing that there is an innate intelligence within all things, (here we are just looking at the body's health possibilities) we then recognize that it has more knowledge of itself than an educated mind does in applying health to it from the outside. This is why it is important to know what the master system of the body is, what structure within the body controls health, and how it does it.

Let's look then at the master system. This system, as I have mentioned, controls and coordinates all the cells, tissues, organs and systems of the body. There's not a lot we can do without its appropriate function. This master system is the nerve system. The nerve system is the innervator of this process of coordination. So it would make sense to make sure that our nerve system is free of interference in its communication so it can clearly coordinate and communicate to all areas in order to create homeostasis (balance), and thus ultimately optimum levels of health expression.

When the nerve system encounters interference, symptoms eventually arise within the body. Firstly, the body adopts different positions in order to maintain health. This might be new for some people; the innate expression within the body is always looking for ways to express health when in a compromised state. When the body adopts postures which aren't familiar, the external expression of health from within will usually be in the guise of pain or a general feeling of discomfort, be it headaches, constipation, stomach upset, leg cramps, numbness, tingling, and so forth. Now, one can choose to mask this pain by thinking that health comes from the outside-in and so take an external substance (usually medication), to take this pain or discomfort away. It's funny — we are brought up in this society where we can have whatever we want at our fingertips and we don't have to do much work for it, and unfortunately we think the same about our health. For example, we can do our banking from home, we can have dinner within seven minutes of getting home via the microwave, we can get from A to B via convenient transport, and we have email for quick contact. Most things within our society today are about instant gratification. It seems many people think that if they aren't feeling whatever it is that they took the medication for in the first place, then they must be healthy. People with symptomatic expression of breast cancer have had it in their body for up to five years prior to it being noticed. People with bowel cancer have often had it in their body for ten years before they display symptoms. I ask you this: during that time when they were asymptomatic, that is they had no known signs or symptoms, were they healthy? The answer, of course, is no. The body gets to a point where it instills symptoms as a means of getting our educated minds to make different decisions, to put our attention onto doing our lives differently. It doesn't give us the gift of discomfort for the benefit of us taking it away through medications and the like. This communication system is one of our greatest gifts.

> THE BODY GETS TO A POINT WHERE IT INSTILLS SYMPTOMS AS A MEANS OF GETTING OUR EDUCATED MINDS TO MAKE DIFFERENT DECISIONS...

Let's take the example of a fridge: it has an internal mechanism for control and it has an electrical source. Let's look at the fridge from the outside. On a daily basis the fridge doesn't change its looks. When we open the door the light goes on and it is assumed the food will be cold. Let's say on this particular day you wake up and open the fridge door and the light is flickering a bit. The food seems fine and the temperature inside still seems cold. The next day you wake up, open the fridge door to find the light is out, the fridge seems rather warm and the food is a bit rancid. What do you do? I would imagine you would check your innervation, the electrical supply. Perhaps there was a power failure the night before and because you were asleep you missed it. The fridge still looks the same on the outside but it isn't until you opened the door that you noticed anything different. It was the power supply, the innervation, the "nerve system" that had changed.

It's the same with us when we wake up in the morning. When we look in the mirror, we see the same person. We don't even realize that changes are taking place internally. The mere fact that by the time we get symptomatic expression there has been approximately a 30% reduction in the function is surely enough to make us sit up and take notice of the ingenious design of the body and what it tries to do for us without us even knowing it. It truly is a humbling experience to acknowledge the internal wisdom that our bodies have.

There are three areas in our life that contribute to a decrease in our health expression. These three areas include thoughts (emotional), trauma (physical), and toxins (chemical) commonly called the 3Ts. We visited these briefly earlier, but in the following chapter I would like to have a look at each in more detail.

The *Vital* Truth

- Health comes from the inside.

- The nerve system is the vehicle through which our expression of health is controlled and coordinated.

- When we have a well-functioning nerve system, with reduced interference we have a greater opportunity of seeing life in balance.

- When we see the perfect order in our life we are able to be grateful for the opportunities that signs and symptoms bring to us.

The *Vital* Questions

- How can your innate intelligence express itself to its optimum level?

- Write about how you can live a more vitalistic life. (A vitalistic approach sees the body as a whole, with the ability to communicate with and heal itself.)

- Most people think of losing some perceived person, place, thing or idea when they are thinking about change. What are you prepared to give up **and** gain as a result of a well-functioning nerve system?

Your notes

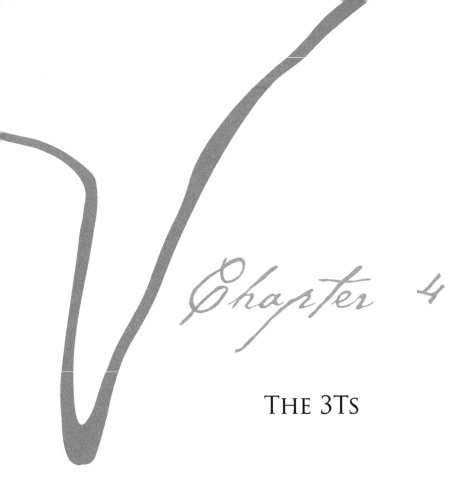

Chapter 4

THE 3TS

"Mental whispers develop dynamic power to reshape matter into what you want… Whatever you believe in intensely, your mind will materialize."

PARAMAHANSA YOGANANDA

There are three main areas in life that affect the body's ability to communicate with itself and outside of itself and which are known as "stressors". These stressors impact our health and contribute to miscommunication within the body. *Stresses*, on the other hand, are how we choose to react to the stressors. Three stressors, which I feel encapsulate most of the areas of life, are referred to as *thoughts*, *trauma* and *toxins*. Coined by D.D. Palmer, the terms describe the emotional, physical and chemical factors which impact our body. Each of these areas can be further broken down into small areas or components that make it more relevant to see where the majority of the impact is upon our life.

When we look at *trauma* (the physical component), there are many examples that we can see which have an impact upon us on a daily basis. Now, remember that by the time we notice symptomatic expressions, there has already been approximately a 30% reduction in the FUNCTION of the body. There is quite a lot that the body can and does put up with in order to create continued expressions of health. The innate intelligence of the body *wants* us to be healthy. It doesn't create postures and diseased states which shall harm us; it creates different postures and communication channels in order to retain a level of health, albeit at a reduced level.

The trauma or physical change that we experience is common and varies in expression. It includes pregnancy, birth, crawling, walking, sport, work, accidents and so forth. Expressions can also be subtle — in most cases we might not be aware that there is reduced communication within our body over a period of time. It's easy to ignore an ache here or there. And here is the crucial point: it's not until we wake up one morning and bend in a particular way, either upon waking or through the course of the day, that our body finally says, "You know what? I need your help right now so I shall provide you with dis-ease, dis-harmony, dis-comfort, or pain — call it what you will — to help you recognize that something in your life needs to be done differently. I'll communicate through the educated mind so that I know you'll be aware of what is happening internally." People choose either to cover the symptoms or address them. What we have done in our lives to date will affect us throughout our lives if we choose to do nothing about it.

It's clear that masking the communication between our innate intelligence and our educated minds will not do us justice over the long term. In fact it will create greater states of dis-ease within the body until such time that the body manifests diseased states and then, in many cases, the symptoms explode.

∽

"The body is a community made up of its innumerable cells or inhabitants."

THOMAS EDISON

∽

The next area to have a look at is *toxins* (the chemical component). This encompasses the air we breathe and the water and food we consume, which has a direct impact on our ability to express optimum health.

Did you know that there are approximately 80% fewer nutrients in the food we consume today compared to that of our grandparents' generation? Find a great organic store within your town or nearby and support the development of this type of farming. Organic and biodynamic farming processes are invaluable to maintaining nutrients in the foods we consume. Most might baulk at the price of this type of food however, like anything, it is based on supply and demand. The more we demand, the cheaper it becomes. "Conventional" foods contain less nutrients and more synthetic ingredients, mainly in the form of additives and preservatives. This isn't new information, but what it does to the body might be new to you.

Toxins can come in all guises including food, pesticides, herbicides, pollution, smoke, drugs, air-conditioning, make-up and gases — the list appears endless. Toxins impact our chemical system (e.g. the endocrine system) on a daily basis.

I have a lady who regularly travels from interstate and comes into the practice to get checked when visiting. She comes in to get checked because she realizes the importance of a balanced system and acknowledges how her body functions at a higher level post-adjustment. She initially came into the practice because she was having concerns about her sporadic menstrual cycle. The day following each adjustment, her menstrual cycle resumes. Adjustments to the master system of the body — the nerve system — affect the chemical system of the body. This lady is a great example of this.

Are the changes in the body so subtle that sometimes you don't even know they are happening? The body, in all its wisdom, created a communication system that is not separate from itself. It communicates internally with all parts of us to create optimum levels of health expression. We *can* live a life of limitless possibility and endless potential if we choose to do so.

"We are what we think. All that we are arises with our thoughts. With our thoughts we make the world."

THE DHAMMAPADA

Our *thoughts* (the emotional component) carry tremendous power. Many people now say that our thoughts create our reality and I was certainly presented with many opportunities to put this belief into practice as I was going through college. When I was in 4th trimester (second year) there was an exceedingly generous scholarship on offer. It was a leadership scholarship and only given to two people in the class. There were around 140 students in our class — small compared to some at 220. The recipient was given access to the "Vogt Leadership Society". With only ten students at any one time in the Society, it was formed to provide up-and-coming students in the profession with the opportunity to develop their leadership skills in the understanding that those selected would do great things within and outside of the profession. Only five students are nominated and upon nomination there are seven rounds of interviews and an essay to write. I remember when my husband and I both received a letter stating nomination. From that day I envisioned myself with every interviewer in every possible situation and going through all the possible questions. I even wrote down the benefits and the drawbacks to receiving the scholarship and the benefits and drawbacks to one of us receiving the scholarship, should just one of us be the recipient. The interview process took three weeks to complete. At the end of that grueling three week period, we were told via letter that we had *both* received the scholarship — a first for a husband and wife who were studying in the same year. I know in my mind the ability to manifest such an honor was because my cause for receiving it was far greater than myself. I had a plan for how the money would be used and a clear vision of what the association with the Society would bring me in the short and long term.

How and what we think of on a daily basis becomes what we attract into our life. If we focus on the pain in our back, the headaches or the sciatic nerve, then this is what we attract into our life. If, however, we choose to recognize ourselves as a self-healing, self-regulating organism with limitless potential to reach optimal health, then fullest expression of this is heightened. It's the metaphysical law of attraction and universal truth that what we focus on becomes our reality. We *can* change our life by changing what we focus on, and then incorporating these thoughts in a balanced way into our lives. It is as simple as that. Live as if what you are asking for has already happened. Look for the benefits and the drawbacks to a given situation and when you are clear as to the balanced perspective of each side and you have reached a state of balance internally, then anything is possible.

> HOW AND WHAT WE THINK OF ON A DAILY BASIS BECOMES WHAT WE ATTRACT INTO OUR LIFE.

The story of my first pregnancy is an incredible example of the power of our thoughts and the truth that our body knows exactly what it is supposed to do at any given time.

When I was pregnant with "Little One", I was still in college studying the remarkable intelligence and nature of the body. I drew strength from the profession's philosophy. However, there was one thing I perceived missing for me: trust that my body could give birth. So I had my doubts about whether there really was intelligence in the body and that the body that forms, grows, and nurtures the baby also had the intelligence to birth the baby. I understood the anatomy and physiology of the body inside out, along with the philosophy at an intellectual level: everything I was taught made sense in theory, but for some reason in practice I found it difficult to acknowledge it.

Every morning upon waking, I would sit having breakfast at our kitchen table and tell the baby it was okay for it to die. I would tell "Little One" I didn't want it; I didn't want to be a mother, I couldn't cope with a baby right now. Did I know that I would have these emotions at the time? No. Yet still something inside me was telling me to tell the baby it was okay to die.

At three months I found myself in the bathroom of a Borders bookstore, crying as I saw large amounts of blood on my underpants. I told my husband we had to go home right away. I was caught between sadness, joy and shock at the self-fulfilling prophecy. It was 3:00 pm in the afternoon. We went around to a friend's place who adjusted me, and it just so happened that the lady filling in to teach the pediatrics program at college was a midwife and was present at our friend's house. After being adjusted and sharing my experience thus far with my friends, my husband and I went home. I lay in bed pondering over what my perceptions had created; the power of my words and mind.

By 10:00 pm that evening movement started to happen: more cramping, contractions and blood loss. I'd been in denial. *Perhaps it's just some bleeding*, I would tell myself. *Lots of women bleed during pregnancy; perhaps this is just what I do.* However, I knew by this time that I was having a miscarriage. At midnight my body started to go into the birthing process. I became exceptionally focused on each contraction as the fetus started to move through the stations of birth. I felt incredible discomfort and pain. I wanted to retreat into another body and return when it was all over. I felt the prostaglandins kick in, my heart rate quicken and my sensitivity increase. No sound could be made. I had to have total quiet.

By 2:00 am it was over. My body and mind collapsed in a heap. I felt guilty, sad, elated, amazed, powerful, and yet so alone. Empty. "Little One" gave me the biggest gift of all: trust in the body — the reason why I am a chiropractor.

The reason why I didn't want to have a baby was the fear of not being able to birth, the fear that my body couldn't do it. "Little One" gave me trust, inner strength, a home birth, no intervention, and acknowledgement that the body knows what to do every time. I didn't go off to hospital to have a D & C. I didn't call a doctor to find out if everything had passed and to find out if I was "okay". I didn't want anything external interrupting the flow I was in with the gift "Little One" had given me — the ultimate gift of trust. I thank you for this gift, "Little One".

My husband took me away the following weekend to relax and reflect at a place called Galena, Iowa. Here I drew, painted and slept. I drew a grateful picture in honor of "Little One". I knew at the time I was painting that nothing is ever missing in our lives; it just changes form. "Little One" is now a beautifully painted picture hanging brightly in our little girl's bedroom.

We went on to have two lovely boys, now four years and two years of age and have recently given birth to a little girl at home which was an unassisted breech. All three were born at home in lovely surrounds. Our eldest was born with Amish midwives, while our second was born at home with my husband and a fellow colleague. All were amazing births which have further cemented for me the gift from "Little One": trust in the body.

The power that made the body has the power to birth and heal the body.

Our thoughts can be extraordinarily insightful if we are willing to look at the origins of them and where we have them manifest in the body. For example, the sacrum is all about our relationship to our father, the hips are about relationships in general, the lower back is about finances, the spine is about support and stability. The body is able to communicate in many different ways. The type of disease we might be experiencing and where that disease is manifesting itself can tell us a lot about what might be happening in our lives and what we are focusing on if we choose to acknowledge it.

The various bone structures play significant emotional roles, as do organs in the body. For example, anger manifests in the liver; trouble in the gall bladder indicates resentment; the adrenals can let us know about muddled instability, the stomach and spleen about low self esteem — the list is endless. This is another way that the body can communicate with us on a daily basis.

".... The belief system is often the activator of the healing system."

NORMAN COUSINS

"Our thoughts are the currency with which we buy our lives."

KAREN WRIGHT

Jen and her daughter Lucy came in on the recommendation of the child's grandmother whom I had been seeing for some time. Lucy's grandmother had mentioned to me that the child was diagnosed with speech delays and asked if I could take a look at her and see if we could help in any way. I said yes — of course I would be happy to chat with the family and give them my opinion of what might be happening from a chiropractic perspective. Sure enough, Lucy did appear to have some delays in speech and understanding. There was certainly interference to her nerve system. This little girl spoke rarely and when she did there was limited understanding. I explained to Jen, Lucy's mother, what was happening and suggested a time frame for care. Jen was diligent in bringing her in because she understood the value of the care.

Along the way I suggested to Jen she might like to schedule herself for a check and see what might be presenting in her own system, after a number of comments she had made about herself. Now, I knew that tied into Lucy's health expression was the complication of her mother's past and the subsequent circumstances surrounding her birth.

Let's remember the 3Ts: thoughts, trauma and toxins for a moment. Is it possible that this little girl had an emotional component to her health expression? As Jen underwent care I noticed changes in Lucy. Our energy is a sphere: it is all-encompassing. We can track on other events that are happening in our life without consciously knowing it.

Jen was a quiet lady, softly spoken and getting information out of her was difficult at times. I asked her one day if she wanted to do some emotional work to help the body move through and beyond where she was at present, to which she agreed. Now, prior to this emotional work with Jen I had been doing some emotional work with Lucy. Jen had noticed a remarkable change in Lucy's speech, yet was still a little hesitant. I felt there was still something holding Lucy back from fully expressing herself.

When the emotional work with Jen began, so too did the little girl start to shine. It turned out that Lucy's mother had been molested when very young and hadn't shared it with anybody. She had shut down as a result. In doing so she had modeled for her daughter that it is not okay to share your emotions, or even have a voice. Sensing this, the little girl had shut down and chosen not to speak. Jen had unwittingly taught her that when you speak, nobody hears you anyway, so why talk? As the emotional work began to unfold, so too did Lucy. She started to come alive! People could understand her better, loved hearing her talk and were delighted with her progress. See the power of the senses! What we feel energetically is absolutely transferred to others.

Next time you wonder whether your child has a problem, check first inside yourself, as it might just be you who has it. What you do and how you handle the situation or perceived problem is critical to who expresses it. Something

I teach all parents is: what gets suppressed gets expressed and it's usually our children doing it for us.

Thoughts *do* change our physiology. In changing our physiology, we affect components of health within our body. Imagine your favourite food. One thought is all it takes for a cascade of physiological responses to occur and the taste buds to salivate! If one thought can do that, imagine what our thoughts can do on a daily basis when we interact with things we love, like and dislike.

> THOUGHTS DO CHANGE OUR PHYSIOLOGY. IN CHANGING OUR PHYSIOLOGY, WE AFFECT COMPONENTS OF HEALTH WITHIN OUR BODY.

In a study done some time ago, Dr. Masaru Emoto, President of the I.H.M General Institute and a doctor of alternative medicine, decided to explore the effect of music, words and thoughts upon water. I am going to look only here at the words and thought component of his research.

Firstly Dr. Emoto and his team put distilled water in bottles and attached words or sentences such as, "love", "war", "peace", "let's", "must" and "I hate you"/ "I want to kill you" to the outside. What he found under microscope was nothing short of extraordinary. The "love", "peace", and "let's" bottles all contained molecules shaped in beautiful geometrical arrangements that glowed with light. The "I hate you"/"I want to kill you", "war", and "must" bottles had a dull colour and an arrangement of molecules that were odd-shaped like a mesh. As the research concludes: "Water enables us to see the hidden power behind words."

Dr. Emoto also did research in the area of spoken words and thoughts projected on to water. Firstly the people said "Thank you, water," and then "We love you, water," and lastly "We'll take good care of you, water." The people were then asked to send the same message via their thoughts; in other words to say the same messages to themselves whilst thinking of the water. Within three hours, the water was observed under microscope. What was produced was a beautifully balanced crystal. The research concluded that "water tells us it can act as our mirror, that it can reflect human thought; water has the ability to show us what we cannot see." I wonder, through this crystallization process and research, what water is trying to tell us? The conclusion for me with this research is if our thoughts can do that to water, imagine what our thoughts are doing to our body, given that 75%-85% of our body is full of water! What states of health are we creating just by our thoughts alone?[4]

When we look at any moment in our lives, it's important to recognize that there are positives and negatives to *all* situations (remember the scholarship story I told you and how I wrote down the benefits and drawbacks to receiving it). Somebody who has been labeled with "depression" finds both a cost and a benefit to having it. Of course most people wouldn't immediately find a positive in there; they just see the negatives. Yet, positives could include receiving attention, phasing out in the mind, rest, and having things done for them. There are as many positives as there are negatives.

When we have something in our bodies that we want to get away from or get rid of, then the body may well heighten its expression. What our bodies want is for us to accept the expression of the symptoms and work with what we have in order to create greater states of balance and acceptance. When the polarities of a disease or symptomatic expression are accepted, when the positive and negative energies are aligned, balance is sought and concurrently the energy charges emit light and, ultimately, love.

It is important to have these energies in harmony with one another and accept that when we are in a situation where we think something is missing or in a situation where we want the other, we need to avoid the "grass is greener over there" syndrome. When we feel that something is missing, we need to look carefully into the world of our own lives and find where it is, because it shall be there — it just might be, as we have mentioned already, in another transmutable form. We have everything that we need and we get everything provided to us by the universe when we ask for it.

The 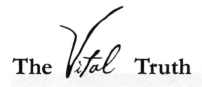 Truth

- There are three stressors which impact our life — D.D. Palmer coined them thoughts, trauma and toxins.

- Each is influenced by the other and each has a direct influence on our ability to create balance in our system.

- When each are acknowledged and seen in the true light in which they are presented, we see the gift which they bring and the opportunities for us to follow.

- When we hear the messages we get an opportunity to change the way we do our lives.

The *Vital* Questions

- What foods do you consume?

- Where is your local organic store?

- What do you spend most of your time thinking about?

- We have the power to change our lives — do you want to?

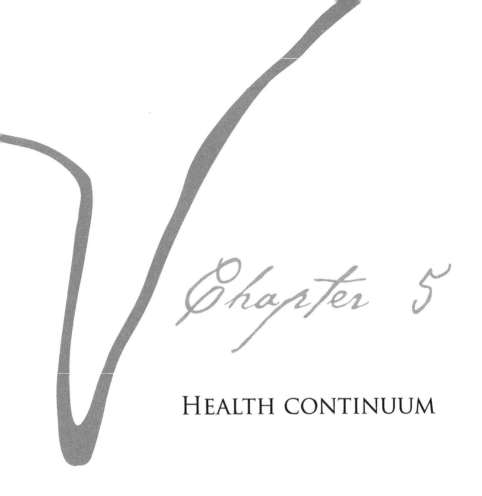

Chapter 5

HEALTH CONTINUUM

"Every truth passes through three stages before it is recognized. In the first it is ridiculed; in the second it is opposed; in the third it is regarded as self-evident."

ARTHUR SCHOPENHAUER 1788 - 1860

Here we shall take a look at the contextual background on health. For over five thousand years there have been two theories about health. We've looked in Chapter one at the atomist/mechanistic point of view. This view breaks down all the structures into physical elements to form basic physical building blocks, so it would look like the following: atoms — molecules — genes — cells — tissues — organs — systems — humans. Then there are the vitalists who think an essential "something" is responsible for organizing matter to keep it functional. The two theories are worlds apart. Either you have a conscious being with a physical expression or you have a complex physical entity that magically gains consciousness.

But what is consciousness? Is it thoughts, feelings, emotions, states of being? Three hundred years ago Newton split the two theories of thought (vitalism and mechanism) and tipped the scales in the direction of the atomists. He did so by postulating "if it is not measurable, than it is a waste of time." Researchers now realise it is exceptionally hard to measure this vitalistic life force, this energy, this "something" in the Western scientific paradigm of experimentation. As a result science, and in many respects, Western thinking began to head in the direction of the atomist.

Instead of a rigid view of "sickness", "health" and "health care", let's consider that health exists on a continuum. This is the idea that people aren't just sick or well, but the idea that our health is continually changing, fluctuating between extremes of ideal and pathological disease. These fluctuations create the continuum [see Diagram 5A].

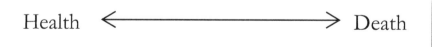

Health $\longleftarrow$ $\longrightarrow$ Death

Diagram 5A: The Health Continuum: a linear perspective

It is important to remove ourselves from the idea that we are either sick or well. We oscillate between all aspects of health, all the time, day in and day out. What is of benefit to the health conscious individual is to view health as a balancing act where homeostasis is the internal mechanism that allows for adaptation to the external environment to take place. So, at times, we might be at either end of the continuum. The important point here is that most of the time we aren't consciously aware of the swings we have along the continuum. The innate intelligence of the internal workings of the body just takes care of it. Our innate intelligence coordinates our health without us consciously having to monitor it day in and day out. There comes a time when the innate intelligence gives the educated mind some awareness and this is when the symptomatic expressions become known to us at a conscious level.

Universal forces as we know them today include, but are not limited to: spiritual, mental, vocational, financial, familial, social, and physical, along with the 3Ts as outlined by D.D. Palmer: thoughts, trauma and toxins. These areas of life are all interrelated and have an impact upon our physiology when we come in contact with them either by cognitive or other means. Our innate intelligence is constantly at work to maintain a balance in the face of the effect of these forces.

Our ability to adapt along this continuum is influenced by the law of homeostasis. Homeostasis, according to the *Macquarie Dictionary*, is the "physiological equilibrium within living creatures involving a balancing of structure, functions and chemical compositions ..." as well as "maintenance of the social equilibrium." By looking at the different levels on the continuum we can see the influence the homeostasis mechanism has on the organism's ability to adapt. It is important to note the 3Ts: thoughts (emotions, social, self), trauma (structure, function) and toxins (chemicals, foods) have an effect on the homeostasis of an individual.

IT IS IMPORTANT TO REMOVE OURSELVES FROM THE IDEA THAT WE ARE EITHER SICK OR WELL.

B.J. Palmer (the developer of Chiropractic) said the vertebral subluxation (meaning *less than light*) is a result of neurological interference and is the number one contributor to the creation of disease within a person. This concept is explained in detail in Chapter seven. The chiropractic message professes that the disease experience is a result of a laden nerve system, where communication with itself is limited and interference heightened. This results in altered states of health expression in all three areas: thoughts, trauma, and toxins.

Now, what would happen if these are impacting an already interfered-with nerve system? The body begins to alter in posture and adjust in function in order to maintain a set level of optimum health: it re-establishes a new balance point. The reason for this is that when we come in contact with things that we are unable to interpret or understand, we change our physiology, which in turn affects how we function and express health on a day-to-day basis. What happens when we watch the news and it's all about war, rape, abductions, ransoms, car accidents, murder, drought, and famine? What happens to the internal workings of our bodies; our innateness? *Our physiology changes depending on our perceptions of the world.* We are seeing, hearing and interpreting a constant stream of one-sided views about what is happening in the world. Our physiology then needs to be equilibrated, balanced, harmonized in order to continue functioning at an optimum level. This happens via the internal workings of the homeostasis mechanism which is a feedback system designed to maintain the balance within. Not only do we balance the internal mechanism of the body; we also balance our perceptual understanding of the world we live in at a micro-level and a macro-level by seeing both sides to a story or situation.

The state of how we are at any given time I refer to as the position on the continuum, illustrating our health at that time. Bear in mind that this state or position is continually changing — the position on the continuum is determined by a number of factors within the body (innate forces) and factors outside the body (universal forces). Hence, a person either adapts to the environment successfully or unsuccessfully.

In Chiropractic, factors within the body and our perceptual understanding of our environment are seen to be the most important in bringing about change in either direction on the continuum. The environment outside can cause health changes, but only if the environmental forces exceed our limits of adaptability. The chiropractor looks inside to find factors that are preventing adaptation to the outside (thoughts, trauma and toxins).

It is also important to note here that chiropractors entertain the idea that the organism becomes stronger or more able to adapt by being exposed to the environment within its limits and not by avoiding it. This holds true for immunity building, which is discussed further in Chapter 20.

If we take a look at the diagram of the continuum [Diagram 5B] which follows, we see four significant sections. Bear in mind there are many states between each of these.

Health & Wellness	Dis-ease	Disease	Death
potential	malfunctions	pathologies	no adaptation

Diagram 5B: Health Continuum with four significant sections

At one end of the continuum we have a high level of health — or optimum wellness — where we are born perfect, with the possibilities to reach our fullest potential and the ability to find optimum balance within the innate genius of the body. All levels are impacted by our thoughts, trauma and toxin realities which we create via the choices we make on a daily basis. The higher our optimum health expression (remember the definition of health from *Dorland's Pocket Medical Dictionary* is "a state of optimum physical, mental and social wellbeing and not necessarily the absence of disease or infirmities"), the better the choices we have made for ourselves.

As we depart from optimum, we venture to functional uneasiness, disharmony or "dis-ease" as D.D. Palmer labeled it. "Dis-ease" simply is the body being uneasy or out of balance with itself. At this level, interference results in changes to the functioning of the body again at either a thought, trauma or toxin level. Messages become misinterpreted as the nerve system becomes compromised.

From dis-ease we travel through to pathology. These are supposed "diseased" states where professions get into naming various conditions which cause people to live according to this belief and hold themselves there — sometimes for the remainder of their lives.

An example of this is cancer. Cancer is nothing more than cells that are doing their own thing. They proliferate because they are not in communication with the tissue intelligence — this is *tissue* intelligence, not innate intelligence. Cancer cells have their own cellular intelligence, and as such care nothing for the good of the whole. Individual cells thrive for themselves, not for others in the collective. It is "all or none" thinking, incorporating one-sided perceptions where people disown a part of what they perceive. This is why the cancer cells are so destructive: they are passive, yet powerful. The cancer cells withhold information from other cells in order to gain their own way. Interestingly, our thoughts, trauma and toxic wellbeing has an impact on how fast these cells proliferate and where they proliferate. Remember the power of an organ is proportional to its own cells communicating with each other. It is *not* a Darwinian theory of survival of the fittest. We only have to look to the cancer cells to understand that this is not the case.

At the other end of the continuum we have death, where adaptation and life no longer exist. The vitality — the life force, that energy, that "something" — is no longer present.

I would like to take a moment here to reframe the *Dorland's Pocket Medical Dictionary* definition of health. When we read the Dorland's definition it is limited to physical, mental and social wellbeing. I have spoken about seven areas of life which have an impact on our ability to reach our optimum health expression: spiritual, mental, vocational, financial, familial, social and physical. Each of these areas is further influenced by each other. They are all interrelated. This is why when we are out of balance in one area we may find balance in another. The key is to find the support and challenge in each of the areas, to raise our awareness to do our life differently, to ask different questions. Evolution, growth and higher levels of understanding are possible with increased awareness about how we do our life. My reframed definition of health is "optimum spiritual, mental, vocational, financial, familial, social and physical wellbeing and not necessarily the absence of disease". This is further represented in the diagrams which follow. [Diagrams 5C – 5F].

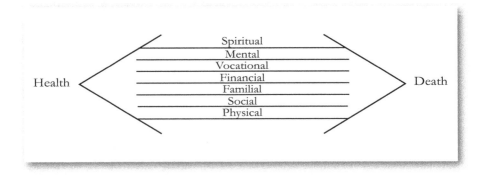

Diagram 5C: Represents the reframed definition of health: multifaceted

As you can see, health is often demonstrated as a simple linear line stretching from optimum health and wellbeing to death. [Diagram 5A] Conceptually, however, the reframed definition of health warrants a new diagrammatical interpretation of health which recognizes that the body's innate wisdom oscillates in a multitude of ways at every point along the continuum so as to represent a wave particle. [Diagram 5D]

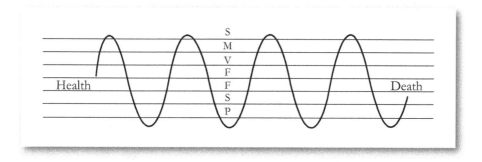

Diagram 5D: Reframed definition of health represented as a wave particle

If you look now at a cross-section of the above wave particle in the diagram which follows [Diagram 5E] as it relates to the new interpretation of health, we see another unique interpretation. Diagram 5E demonstrates how all seven areas are interrelated. This interpretation allows us to see where the polarity in our life may exist. The outer part of the circle contains optimum wellbeing and health expression (100%). The innermost area of the circle contains death (0%). The line in the middle represents the linear balance point for each of the areas. This is where all the areas are aligned and true growth takes place. Most importantly, health *and* disease are necessary for growth and evolution. We don't grow by avoiding disease. It is around us constantly. This is why the balance point lies in the middle as seen in Diagram 5E.

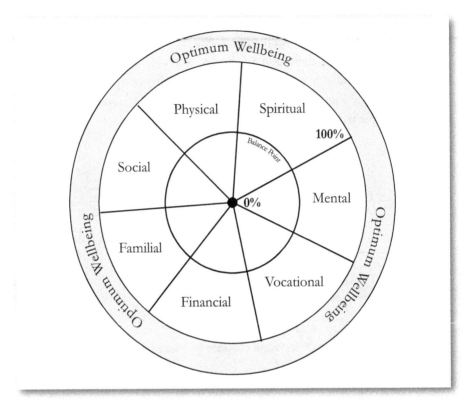

Diagram 5E: Cross-section of a wave particle showing all seven areas of life

On the following diagram [Diagram 5F (A)], plot where you are at present in your life. Once you have plotted all the areas, join up all the dots so you can see the interconnection and the imbalances. See Diagram 5F (B) as an example. In being able to see where the imbalances lie, we can awaken ourselves to asking different questions. One question we might like to ask ourselves is: if this was a tire on our car, what would the ride be like?

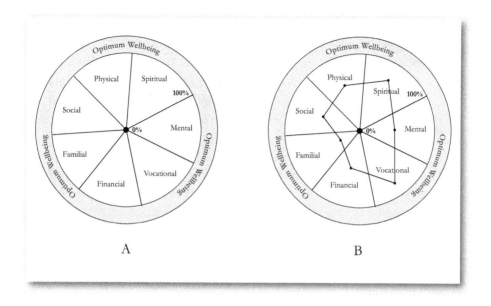

Diagram 5F: (A) Plot your own values on the wheel; (B) An example of where a person's imbalances lie

"The problem with our health care system is that you have to lose your health to enter it."

DR. DEAN BLACK

From the vitalist's perspective comes the model of "innate intelligence", the inborn knowledge that all forms of life possess and express. The innate intelligence has the ability to maintain homeostasis, to maintain balance, which in turn leads to greater function, greater expressions of health and adaptation to the environment. The nerve system is responsible for coordinating all the cells, tissues, organs and systems of the body, thereby enabling maintenance of homeostasis and adaptation to the surrounding environment.

The life force within enables everything to be kept together. The inborn or innate intelligence, the matter (our physical body through which force is expressed) and the force (required to unite intelligence and matter), is known as the Triune of Life. Within this triune is the postulation that energy exists in waves which have a physical expression. Therefore if we only look for physical causes and realities then we are missing out on the majority of what is life – movement and energy!

In 1927 a gentleman called R.W. Stephenson wrote the 33 principles of Chiropractic, listed in full at the end of this book. The first principle is known as the Major Premise and states: "A universal intelligence is in all matter and continually gives to it all its properties and actions, thus maintaining it in existence." Health care under the medical model does not share this theoretical underpinning.

It is important to respect this innate intelligence and accept that ALL parts of the body were designed with specific functions in mind. Removing parts of the body disrupts the whole system and does not necessarily restore health. For example, research now tells us the appendix has a vital function in immunity. When the appendix is removed, disruption occurs to the immune system, creating increased functional strain on other organs which are now required to support its function.

I would like to share with you the following piece written by my husband Randall to emphasize where people get caught in the dogma around illness:

A virus in your nose is called a runny nose.

The same virus in your nose and head is called a cold.

The same virus in your nose, head and throat is called a cold with a sore throat.

The same virus in your bronchi is called bronchitis.

The same virus in your bronchioles is called bronchiolitis.

The same virus in your aveoli or deep in your lungs is called pneumonia.

The virus is exactly the same; however we tend to jump up and down when we hear pneumonia or bronchiolitis (what's that?) as opposed to a runny nose. The reason someone got pneumonia from the same virus that someone got a runny nose is due to the state of health of the person in the first place. In our practice I ask people to ask themselves: what is this health expression telling me about my health, and therefore my physical, chemical and emotional reality right now? Ask yourself: where am I out of balance in my life?

"Health is not a condition of matter, but of mind."

MARY BAKER EDDY

I have already defined and reframed the *Dorland's Pocket Medical Dictionary* definition of health, which by the way is also used by the World Health Organization. Both of these definitions have nothing to do with symptoms — being "in" or "out" of pain. In knowing and understanding this interpretation of health, let's take a look at where health comes from.

Ill-health does not always involve pain. We can have pain with no symptoms and symptoms without pain. It's about balance and reaching our full potential in all seven areas of life. Alternatively to Dorland's, *Webster's Dictionary*, on the other hand, focuses on function. It says "health is a state where parts of the body are functioning properly all the time." Webster's tells us exactly how to be healthy, noting that health is a state of wholeness in which all the organs are functioning 100% of the time. Like Dorland's, it says that when everything is functioning in a coordinated manner, we are able to express health to an optimum level.

In understanding health, we see a nerve system which provides a continuum of function and coordination, which enables adaptation to our environment and homeostasis to be reached.

If we have a nerve system functioning 100% of the time, then we have a greater ability to be able to reach optimal states of spiritual, mental, vocational, familial, financial, social and physical wellbeing, thereby enabling health to be expressed.

The chiropractic profession has spent over a century perfecting the philosophy, science and art of the adjustment to aid the body in its adaptation to the internal and external forces acting on it. Imagine if the population of the world lived with adjusted nerve systems. Imagine living with less internal stress and functioning at optimum levels of health. Imagine if we did this for a day and then two days, a week, a month and then a year. Now wouldn't that six o'clock news look different? More balanced, perhaps?

The *Vital* Truth

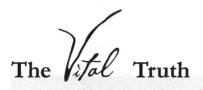

- Health exists on a continuum.

- We are never in one place on the continuum for long; we oscillate between points.

- We can have pain with no disease and disease with no pain.

- Health is about reaching optimum spiritual, mental, vocational, financial, familial, social and physical wellbeing and not necessarily the absence of disease or infirmity.

- Disease is a necessary part of our evolution.

The *Vital* Questions

- Where do you currently sit on the health continuum?

- What are the true indicators of health?

- Do you oscillate around a particular point on the continuum?

- Where is your body challenged in its function? (systems, glands, organs etc.)

- Fill in the Seven areas of Life circle [Diagram 5F (A)] to see where you are experiencing imbalances.

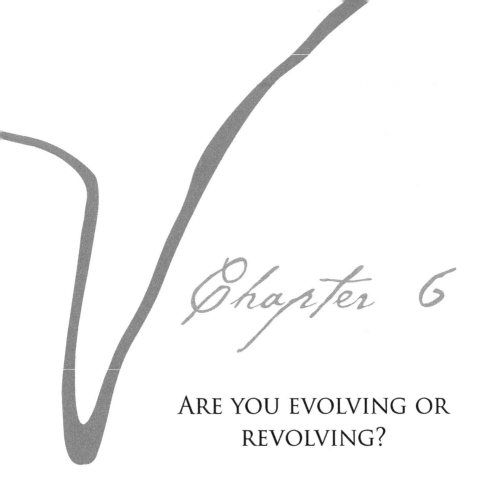

ARE YOU EVOLVING OR REVOLVING?

"Thousands and thousands of people have studied
disease. Almost no one has studied health."

ADELLE DAVIS

We were born to be healthy. The innate wisdom of the unborn child knows what to do and how to express health on the inside, provided there is no interference to this communication and inner knowing. Once in the physical world the child, as it develops through life, is exposed to a number of different stressors. We mentioned these earlier as the 3Ts: *thoughts, trauma* and *toxins,* which over a lifetime have an impact on the communication system of the body. They gradually and often imperceptibly have both a deconstructive and constructive effect on the body's communication system. However, when the deconstructive forces (universal) are greater than the constructive (innate) forces, the body starts to get symptomatic expression [Diagram 6A].

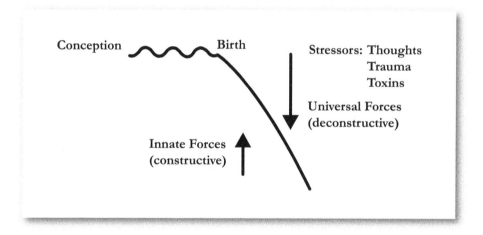

Diagram 6A: An illustration of the forces acting upon us

So we have universal forces bearing down upon us, deconstructing us, and the innate forces internally trying to construct us. These two opposing forces are absolutely necessary for the growth of the body over time. When the deconstructive forces are greater than the constructive forces, we generally see less adaptation to the external world and more symptoms [Diagram 6B].

When we have symptomatic expression, we've crossed the line [Diagram 6B]. That's why we call this "living below the line", and the line is at a different level for everybody, depending on how much of an impact the 3Ts have had on our lives.

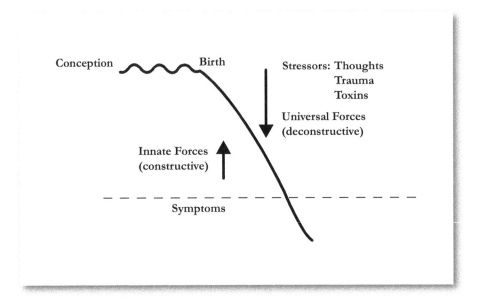

Diagram 6B: Crossing the line to symptomatic expression

When we have symptomatic expression, it's a result of the outside forces being greater than the internal forces. The homeostasis feedback mechanism is more challenged in its response and ultimately its search for balance within the internal world. You find it harder to adapt to the external environment. When adaptation is challenged, you may display symptomatic expression.

Most people take medications of some sort when we have symptomatic expression in order to take the perceived pain or symptom away. This generally takes us *above* the line [Diagram 6C].

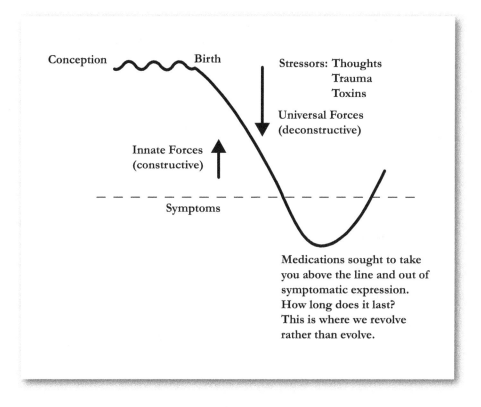

Conception — Birth

Stressors: Thoughts
       Trauma
       Toxins

Universal Forces
(deconstructive)

Innate Forces
(constructive)

Symptoms

Medications sought to take
you above the line and out of
symptomatic expression.
How long does it last?
This is where we revolve
rather than evolve.

Diagram 6C: Moving above the line via an outside-in approach to health

What would we do now that we are sitting above the line with no perceived symptoms due to medications and the like? Well, in the mechanistic model, we would think we were healthy again because we have no pain. Remember, however, that it has taken time for these symptoms to awaken us and appear at a conscious level. I believe the majority of the population chooses to live around this line. This is the area where we are revolving rather than evolving. We have the possibility of looking at health differently at this level and, in fact, the symptoms often take us to all and sundry in our search for greater meaning about what is happening internally. If we do embrace the true understanding of what our bodies are telling us, and awaken ourselves to the possibilities of what lies ahead, then we can begin to evolve to new understandings and perceptions, both in our lives and in the lives of those around us. Eventually, however it gets to a stage where the revolving door of medications we're taking to get us "above the line" and into perceived health aren't working any more. So what do we do? Usually we take stronger and stronger medications in order to keep ourselves "above the line"; we revolve around this point [Diagram 6D].

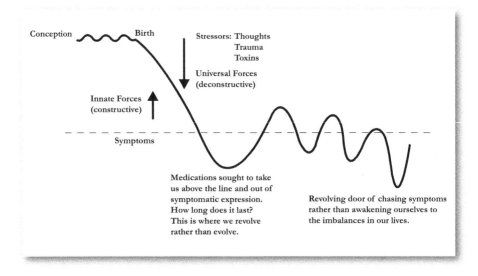

Diagram 6D: The revolving door of medications

Eventually we take other medications to help alleviate the symptoms from the first medications we were consuming, and so end up taking a plethora of medications to counteract the original prescriptions. Out of habit, fear, or lack of understanding, many of us don't awaken ourselves to the imbalances we have in our lives and would rather mask the pain then make the change.

It has been my observation that when we aren't prepared to change our lives in order to heal and grow, it is because we're getting some perceived benefit out of the situation. There are positives and negatives to each situation and to each change. What I have noticed is that often in our quest for growth, healing and change, we tend to focus on the fear of losing something rather than on the possibilities of gaining something. In this light, we rarely see that there are just as many benefits as there are perceived drawbacks to the change or the situation. When we *do* see the situation in balance, we will be liberated in some way — released from burdens such as guilt, pain, or lopsided illusions that we were carrying about an experience or a situation as we have understood it.

If we go back now to looking at the diagram, we see that eventually, after taking medication after medication, people realise that nothing works any more [Diagram 6E].

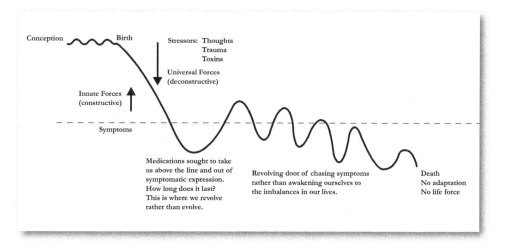

Diagram 6E: No adaptation

We see that more is not better and we then often either resort to invasive methods like surgery or give up, holding an unyielding belief that nothing can help us. If you say "nothing can help me" often enough to yourself and the community then you manifest just that — you create it. In this self-fulfilling prophecy nobody will be able to help you. When a person comes into the practice for an initial consultation and they say "I am not sure if you can help; I have had this for so long and I've tried everything," they often haven't ticked that they have seen a chiropractor before, and I tell them that they *haven't* tried everything. I also point out that if they thought nothing could be done, then why try at all? Usually they reply that they are tired of living the way they are.

After beginning to undergo chiropractic care, people soon realise the power of their body and begin to see life in a different light. The biggest change I initially see in people is the difference in their mindsets. Their perception of their life is altered. They begin to see the benefits from where they are at present and, more importantly, they are awakened to the limitless possibilities which lie ahead.

When people start to see the limitless possibilities, they tend to want more of what they are receiving. In this light and with the education I provide for people to be informed about the neurological interference to the body and what that sets up for them in their lifetime, people start to see the benefits in having regular adjustments. Some come in weekly for the rest of their lives, some monthly and others visit quarterly. It all depends on what the body requires at the time in order to create states of balance internally, whilst enabling challenges externally. It is much like the musician who plays a gig every Saturday night — he won't only tune his guitar once a week. He'll most probably tune it each time he sits down to rehearse. He understands the attention to detail and can hear the tone it makes when it is in balance.

Sue brought her son in to get checked some time ago now. I asked the young boy, James, what it was that he loved to do in his life. His inspiration was playing rugby. That's all he wanted to do — watch it, play it, train in it, read about it. He was inspired by rugby. His mother wanted to get him checked and adjusted because she had been told he had a promising future in the sport and she wanted him to excel. A friend had told her about chiropractic and the internal communication system and how it had benefited her daughter, so she thought she would investigate further. James was due to try out for the state under 15s' team in the following few months. I explained to James about the nerve system and how the internal communication system functions. Once I had completed the examination and mapped out a schedule of care, Sue turned around and said, "That all sounds great — I'll schedule with the front desk to bring him in every Monday after his weekend game on Saturdays."

"No," I replied. "Bring him in on Fridays to ensure his system is communicating with itself at the most optimum level prior to him playing on the Saturday — then if he is challenged during the game on the weekends you can bring him on the Monday." Sue looked at me as if she had had an epiphany. The lights went on and she got it. It wasn't long before the whole family was under care — all seven of them!

If Michael Schumacher was about to perform in the Formula 1 Grand Prix, do you think he would say to his pit crew, "You know, let's not worry about tuning the car now. I'm about to go out and race and the car's going to get challenged anyway, so let's just check it when I get back." Of course he wouldn't. He wants that car as finely tuned and in coordination with itself as he can get it for the purpose of it performing at an optimum level. He wants to perform at his best and in order to do that he requires a car that is optimally tuned. Wouldn't you want that for your body when the mechanism we have inside of us is far greater than the minds that can make a Formula 1 car?

People who choose to live in this "tuned up" way reach optimum levels of health expression in their lives. These people are attracted to the wellness model of care. These people move and live beyond the line. They reach for greater understanding in all areas of their life [Diagram 6F].

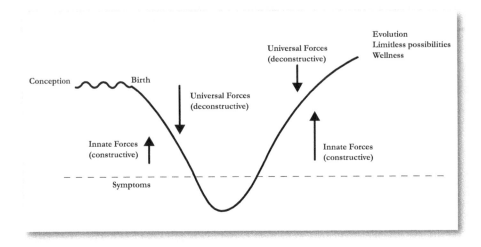

Diagram 6F: Attaining wellness and limitless possibilities

Wellness, as defined by the USA National Wellness Association, is "an active process of becoming aware of and making choices toward a more successful existence." We can choose to accept greater responsibility in all areas of life: spiritual, mental, vocational, financial, familial, social and physical. It starts with the conscious decision to assume responsibility for our lives, to adopt a mindset towards this change and so enable the inception of key principles which lead to a high level of wellbeing and life satisfaction. Wouldn't you rather evolve than revolve?

The 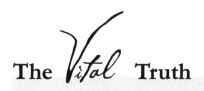 Truth

- There are three distinct levels on our way to optimum health expression. If we choose to live in mediocrity, we walk a path where masking symptoms enables us to move forward in life, but with limitation.

- Those of us who seek wellness care are accessing possibilities in our lives all the time and understand the divine perfection in every circumstance. We see the balance that life brings, and in so doing reach greater understanding in our lives and the lives of those around us.

- If we see the support and challenge in each situation, we are more able to evolve to the next level of support and challenge in our lives, rather than revolve around some arbitrary point in our health.

The Vital Questions

- Do you take medication after medication in order to mask the symptoms, rather than awaken yourself to the possibilities which are available to you by making just one change in your life?

- How can you change your current perceptions so that you start to evolve rather than revolve?

- Where are you choosing to live at present? Below the line, at the line or beyond the line?

- Where would you like to live in the future? Are you willing to do what it takes to get there?

- Write down at least 25 ways in which you can listen to your internal communication system and make the necessary changes in your life.

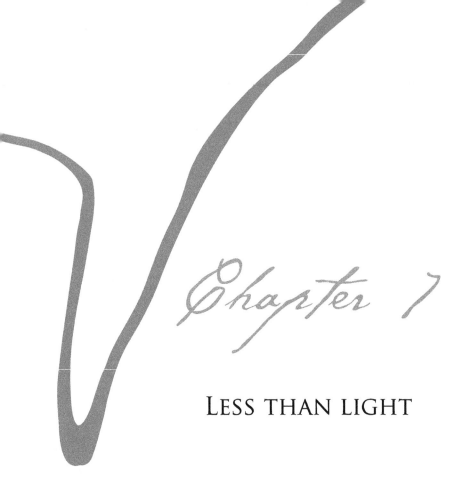

Chapter 7

LESS THAN LIGHT

"We can easily forgive the child who is afraid of the dark.
The real tragedy of life is when men are afraid of the
light."

PLATO

When discussing the innate wisdom of the body, it is important to acknowledge the ingenious design of the nerve system. Changes within the body via physical, chemical or emotional stressors cause changes in the nerve system — the communication system of the body — in order to maximize its conscious communication with you. These changes in the communication system can come via pain, numbness, soreness, coughs or disease. The list is almost endless as to what the mind and the body can create in order to communicate with you. Either, both or all of the three areas — physical, chemical or emotional — together create changes in the homeostasis (balance) feedback mechanism.

These changes within the communication system of the body (the nervous system) are known to the chiropractic community as subluxations: *Sub* meaning "less than", *lux* being "light" and *ation* being "a condition of". Subluxation means *a condition of less light*. When interruption occurs to this delicate system, the body expresses less than light. It expresses darkness, dis-harmony, dis-eased states of health expression where we live in a state of disequilibrium and view life in a lopsided way. You haven't lost health; you just have less expression of it. Health is still stored inside you as potential energy ready to be expressed when the communication is restored.

Energy has two sides: a positive and a negative charge. What then will balance out the darkness, the "less than light" situation in the body, the disharmony, and the dis-ease? Light. The opposite of darkness is light. To remove darkness, you turn on the light.

Chiropractors are qualified to detect and correct subluxations in order to restore the light to the body via the nerve system. Chiropractors are qualified in correcting the subluxations for the purpose of helping the body to help itself adapt to its environment and express health to its optimum level.

On a daily basis, we are unaware of what is happening in our bodies. Let's take the feet as an example. We have no awareness of the soles of our feet until somebody says "how are the soles of your feet doing?" We innately are unsure until someone asks a question which puts our attention there or until something happens to one or both of them, such as getting a stone in our shoe. This feedback mechanism is not occurring via the educated mind. It is the innate intelligence, the wisdom of the internal communication system, that is allowing our body to notice the educated mind and the stone in our shoe.

What about liver cirrhosis? The educated mind doesn't know we have it. The innate intelligence of the body is taking care of it. The drinking causes the innate intelligence to work harder. The innate intelligence is not wired to tell us how the inside is doing. For example, what happens when we chew and then swallow a piece of apple? Once the apple is in the mouth, the salivary glands are activated and particular enzymes are released in order to help digest the food. In actuality the salivary glands become activated just prior to the food being consumed. They are initiated via the thought process of the apple coming into the mouth. Once chewed, the apple is swallowed. We are aware of these two processes because we can feel them. Once the apple has passed the epiglottis and moves into the esophagus it is out of our consciousness.

Once the apple reaches the stomach there is no awareness of the acid being released and of the churning occurring to digest the apple. We are unable to consciously know when it then moves to the duodenum, small intestines, large intestines and lastly rectum. However, research via the educated mind gives us an idea of the digestion process. The innate intelligence of the body monitors its progress from top to tail. If, however, the innate intelligence chooses to have outside assistance, a consciousness is gained by us to change our behaviors and perceptions of the world we live in. The innate intelligence does this via feedback to the educated mind, providing us with the awareness to make the necessary changes. This feedback occurs via subluxations — areas of the body which express less than light — and can occur via the changes in the 3Ts: thoughts, trauma and toxins (emotional, physical, chemical) to awaken us to the imbalances in our lives.

The innate intelligence of the body prefers not to use the educated mind to do the internal healing on an everyday basis. Bearing this in mind, we can do one of two things: wait until we feel disharmony within the body, or have our communication system — our nervous system — adjusted regularly, thereby enabling the innate intelligence of our body to work at its optimum level.

Symptoms are an internal change in the balance mechanism (homeostasis) by which we are challenged. We often don't embrace this communication from the body because it requires us to look at ourselves. What is of concern is that we don't notice anything is wrong until it occurs. So here would be the ideal approach: engage in regular adjustments so we have a system which can communicate with itself, which in turn enables growth and optimum states of function to occur. If signs and symptoms do occur, we are then better able to embrace them and see the support *and* challenge in what they provide, and make the necessary changes in our lives to adjust to the incoming messages from the innate intelligence.

There exists two sides to everything. Just as we have said energy has a positive and negative, so too do our emotions in life. Depression, elation; happy, sad; success and failure, to name just a few. The balance is everywhere. However if we continue to take medications and mask the beauty of what our body is saying to us, we live in the dark for long periods. Would you prefer to live in the light with occasional darkness, or darkness with occasional light? We have the possibility of living a life full of potential and optimal health expression.

The *Vital* Truth

- When we have symptoms, we are motivated into action. Most of us prefer not to live with the perceived inconvenience of signs and symptoms.

- Prevention kicks in the day after something has occurred.

- Remember: having no symptoms doesn't mean you are healthy, and having symptoms doesn't mean you are sick!

- In order for your body to function at its peak, it must be able to communicate with itself.

- The communication of the body is housed in the nervous system.

- When disruption to the communication system takes place it is called a subluxation: a condition of less than light.

- As Plato said "…the real tragedy of life is when men are afraid of the light."

- Clear your subluxations regularly and clear the way to live in the light.

The 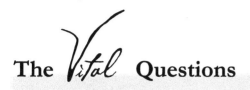 Questions

- Write about seven ways in which you can change your life.

- If reaching your fullest potential in life is now becoming a priority, then what would your wildest dreams look like?

- Do you want an internal communication system which can heal optimally, without you consciously knowing what it is doing?

- Are you waiting until you have signs and symptoms before you seek help in reaching new found levels of optimum health expression?

- How do you know you are healthy?

- Does it make sense to you to get your nerve system checked, to get your "house" in order?

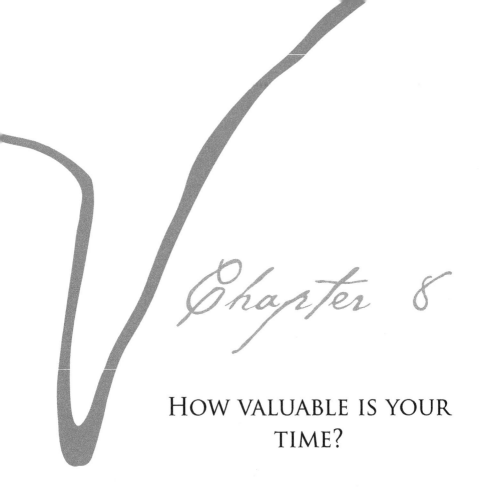

Chapter 8

HOW VALUABLE IS YOUR TIME?

"There are three great physicians: Time, Nature, Patience."

CHINESE PROVERB

Every process we go through requires time. Whether it is the aging process, the birth of a child, job promotions, graduating, or learning new skills like walking, talking or riding a bike. Reaching new milestones and new levels in understanding takes time. I imagine we all agree with this so much so that we place a value on it. For instance, time is money and medals, every second counts, there's no time to waste, if we don't go now we won't have time, if it's not there in 30 minutes it's free! People even get impatient in the drive-through for the "fast food". Most people want instant gratification and immediate results, just like the instant microwave dinner that is "cooked" in one minute.

So many things take time. Cooking a turkey at Christmas takes three or four hours, pregnancy takes nine months and career achievements take time. Yet when it comes to our bodies we seem to be a lot less tolerant of the process of time. The innate time of your body is vastly different to the man-made time of "I want it done yesterday."

Anything quick, artificial, cheap, or that has an easy option to it will probably only give you short term results and may have an altered long-term effect on your body.

Paradox:

"Those who spend little time on their health have little time."

Let's look at the nervous system. When we have a sprained ankle, we generally stay off it. When we break our arm or leg, it is usually put in plaster and immobilized. Is it because the arms and legs are so imperative to daily activities that we notice it more when something is amiss? When plaster is applied to a fracture, the fracture is immobilized and we could be out of pain within days.

Does that mean that we can remove the plaster and start using the arm or leg again? Certainly not. The cast reminds us that we have time left in the healing process. A scab on the skin reminds us that the healing process is still taking place. But what is there to remind us that the nervous system is regaining its optimum health expression? Nothing. This is the risk we get into when we think that because there is no scab or cast, and now no symptoms, we must be "healthy" and healed.

It has been my observation that we tend to follow the recommendations outlined to us for healing when it is an extremity such as the appendicular skeleton that is symptomatically expressing in some way and preventing us from undertaking certain activities. Yet we seem to easily compromise the central aspects of the body, the axial skeleton. In my observation small indicators of pain such as a niggle, headache, or a dull ache are ignored until we are unable to bear it any longer. We then seek care, often entertaining unrealistic expectations about the healing process. When we think in this way, we live in the allopathic paradigm where something from the outside supposedly takes care of the inside. Sometimes we want change as soon as possible, and we are usually unwilling to change any of our lives (physically, chemically or emotionally) in order to help the body to help itself in the healing it can do. People often want change at all costs, and they invariably want it rectified yesterday.

When people come into the practice, one of the most important pieces of information I share with them is the *initial* tissue healing time of the body, which generally takes 6-8 weeks. Even though they may experience a reduction in their symptomatic expression, that doesn't mean they are healed and healthy. All it means is that the symptoms are reduced and the body is now able to communicate with itself more clearly. The body is still on its journey to healing, but is not yet healed. However, what if we changed the emotional (thought) and chemical (toxin) realities as well and not just the physical (trauma)?

IN MY OBSERVATION SMALL INDICATORS OF PAIN SUCH AS A NIGGLE, HEADACHE, OR A DULL ACHE ARE IGNORED UNTIL WE ARE UNABLE TO BEAR IT ANY LONGER.

George was eight when he came into the office with his parents who were beside themselves, trying to work out how to alleviate the severe constipation their son had been experiencing for two-and-a-half weeks. They had tried all and sundry with little success. George described passing a stool as very painful. At this stage George was trying to hold on rather than experience the pain of attempting to go to the bathroom.

Upon receiving a series of physical adjustments, he started to change his internal environment and his body was able to coordinate the peristaltic movement to propel the fecal material through the intestinal system. The adjustments changed his life. No longer was he straining to pass a stool nor having the feeling of being bound up. An emotional technique used in the practice was also run to help the family deal with any emotional issues felt to be binding him up. George had recently changed schools and a new sibling had been introduced to the family. His parents found a huge relief when they were asked certain questions about his life to date. After the first adjustment, young George was able to pass a stool. His body, post-adjustment, was now coordinating a series of events in order to create greater states of health. The emotional issues brought to the surface were able to be integrated for the parents and you could see George's body relax into a feeling of "somebody now knows what I have been experiencing."

The chemical component was also discussed, which his parents were also dedicated to changing. George's life had changed as a result of this interaction. On subsequent visits to the office George found himself racing to the toilet before getting adjusted: his body knew how the adjustment would be received and his innate intelligence was allowing him to reach new states in his health expression at all levels.

Now, George and his parents could have decided after one successful trip to the bathroom that he no longer needed to work on this area of his health expression. Yet he and his parents realized that it takes time to readjust the internal system and, likewise, acknowledged they needed to invest time into this process. *This young man still receives chiropractic care today* — his family recognizes that the adjustment isn't about alleviating symptoms from the body in order to "feel better" but rather allowing your life to be the best it can be in all areas. He's now a 16-year-old budding sports professional, and upon completion of school wants to make a go of it on the professional circuit.

The emotional component of healing is an interesting process for a lot of people. Some people, although wishing to get well, actually find they benefit from where they are in their present situation. Making a decision between the supposed benefits they receive from their current situation, and the genuine benefit that comes with having each system in their body functioning at its optimum level is a challenge for them. Some want change but are too scared to embrace the new self to truly see what they may gain from the change. Most only see the loss.

All processes in life take time — whether a flower is blossoming, the sun is rising, a storm is brewing, or tissue is healing. With time comes clarity and perspective — at all levels: physical, chemical and emotional.

The story of a young man called John who came in to see me some years ago illustrates the understanding for a long-term perspective in reaching new levels of health.

I had only been in practice a short while when John's sister, Susan, came in to see me. Susan was having continual headaches at the time and thought she would give Chiropractic a go. As she sat in the corner of the room and described the headaches to me, it was obvious from her body language that she was reserved and unsure about finding a better expression of health. She explained she felt hesitant at the thought of going to a chiropractor and had reservations around her own internal ability to heal. Her goal in life was to be a surgeon. "We'll certainly have some interesting conversations along the way!" I said. After a series of adjustments, Susan was functioning better within herself and she noticed the first thing to change was her perceptions about life. She shared with me she was making different decisions and as a result gaining different outcomes. She had noticed her headaches had subsided from every day to a couple of times per week and eventually to the occasional one every few months. She had had a remarkable change in her health expression.

On one particular visit, Susan asked me if I could help her brother. I asked her what challenges he was facing in his life and she explained he was challenged genetically which prevented him from doing a lot of things. On top of this, Susan said he had growth and speech delays. In fact, John

> ALL PROCESSES IN LIFE TAKE TIME ... WITH TIME COMES CLARITY AND PERSPECTIVE — AT ALL LEVELS: PHYSICAL, CHEMICAL AND EMOTIONAL.

didn't speak at all. "How about we check him and see what we come up with?" I suggested. I did point out to Susan I wasn't sure how he would respond, because I didn't have a crystal ball. However I knew one thing for sure and that is there is a perfect human being living inside him. We would just need to help him to help himself to shine.

John was booked in for an initial consultation and arrived with Susan and their mother, Kate. When I entered the adjustment room I saw John sitting in the corner with his body well and truly slumped forward. As we chatted I put together a case history from Kate and his sister about his life thus far. John was far from responding to the neurological tests I carried out, and following instructions was a challenge for him. John, his mother and sister taught me some sign language which we used to communicate for some time.

On one particular visit I asked John's mother what was inspiring to him. She looked at me with a blank stare. "Everybody has a genius inside of them," I explained, "and something that inspires them. What is John's?" I asked her how he filled his time and what he loved to do.

"He loves animals, birds, insects, plants of any kind," said Kate. She recounted a story for me about his amazing connection with birds. They were down at the lake watching their daughter row on a Sunday afternoon. As John's parents sat in the park by the lake watching their daughter, they suddenly noticed John wasn't by their side. Within the blink of an eye he'd gone to the water's edge. What was more remarkable was what he was doing — John had approached a pelican and was sitting next to it, chatting, with his arm around its body. John's gift is in his energy which vibrates and resonates with birds, animals, insects, and plants — nature. He has a gift like none other that I have met.

After a few adjustments incorporating the areas of the 3Ts (thoughts, trauma and toxins), I began to see changes in him. John was more upright in his physical presence and was able to respond to some instructions.

The family was diligent about care; they never missed an adjustment and would bring him back if another check was required later in the week. They knew the process would take time and were prepared to stick at the outlined schedule of care for him. After only a few weeks of care his mother was starting to notice remarkable changes, so much so that she scheduled herself for an initial consultation and subsequently regular care. It wasn't long after that when John's father was coming in for regular care as well.

After two months of continued diligent care by his parents and sister in all three areas — thoughts, trauma, toxins — we all saw incredible life-changing results. One day Kate excitedly rang me and recounted what had taken place the night before: they'd been watching TV and as she flicked through the channels John turned to her and as plain as day said, "Mum, I was watching Channel 21!" Tears rolled down my face as I was humbled by the sheer genius of the innate workings of the body. When all others had given up on John's ability to heal, change and integrate into society, I didn't. I knew there was a genius inside. Our bodies are truly intelligent. I am grateful for having witnessed and been a part of the opportunity to help switch on someone's light.

Years later, John and his family are still under chiropractic care. His body now functions at a higher level and he is certainly speaking more clearly. John went on to win a tuition scholarship at his school in his second-last year. Last year he graduated from school and now works at the local nursery. His sister, Susan, is now at Chiropractic College and looks forward to switching on the light in other people's lives.

A lot of people had given up on John and told the family they'd have to accept the way he was, probably for the rest of his life. I know, however, that the power that made the body has the ability to heal the body. It just may take some time.

Everybody has a gift, if we choose to look.

The *Vital* Truth

- Processes take time.

- When the body is ready to receive new insights and the internal balance is present, then change and understanding can be rapid.

- As the Paradox says "Those who spend little time on their health have little time." Take the time to make the changes in your life to see what you will gain from the experience, rather than what you will lose.

- We are constantly constructing and deconstructing our bodies. In order to reach new levels of understanding and search for new support and challenges, we must be prepared to let go of the old to embrace the new.

The *Vital* Questions

- What is your gift?

- What inspires you?

- How would you like to share your inspiration with the world?

- Where in your life do you perceive yourself to be lacking time?

- Are there any areas (spiritual, mental, vocational, familial, financial, social, and physical) in your life where you want instant gratification?

- Consider any benefits you might be receiving from your current position on the health continuum, and ask yourself whether you'd like to move towards a more optimal expression of health.

~

"Those who spend little time on their health have little time."

~

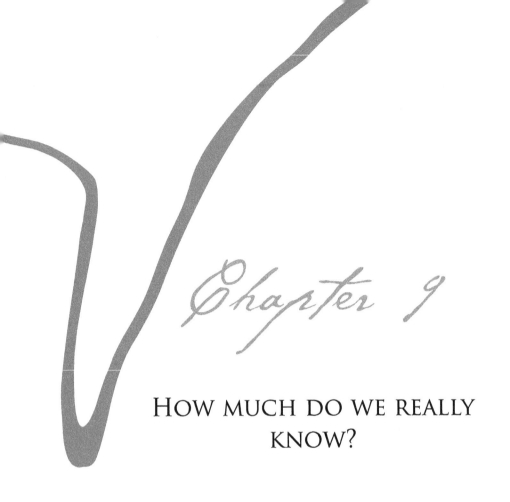

Chapter 9

HOW MUCH DO WE REALLY KNOW?

"I am the wisest man alive, for I know one thing, and that is that I know nothing."

SOCRATES

My greater understanding of life and the thirst for how it operates came when I was 13 years old. I was playing high level tennis at the time and my coach, Craig, wanted to enrol me for junior Wimbledon. Each afternoon I'd go to my grandparent's place to train. And train I did. I would be there for hours after school hitting the balls back and forth with Craig. I usually walked home afterwards but on one particular day Dad had arrived to collect me on his way home from work. As he walked in the gate of his parents' place, he did as he always did. He walked straight to the balcony and leant over the side to watch with what seemed like mesmerized eyes. He would put in his comments as he watched from the "stand" — comments such as "You've got a great swing on you!" I used to feel happy at the acknowledgment, whilst at the same time finding it hard to give it to myself that, yes, perhaps I was a good tennis player. Good, however, wasn't enough — I had to be excellent. Perfect.

On completion of the training for the day I shared with Dad on the way home in the car the possibility of playing at junior Wimbledon. I said that Craig thought I was ready but somehow I didn't feel ready inside. I told Dad how scared I was at the thought of it. As Dad drove the car home he leant towards me with his arm on the middle console and pointed his finger. He said, "Sarah, you can be anything you want to be if you put your mind to it." This was a profound turning point in my life and it was only recently that I shared this story with friends and family at his 70th birthday. He taught me I could indeed do anything and my only limitation was the limitation I chose to place on myself.

As the words stuck like glue I spent many a night and day wondering what the statement "if I put my mind to it" actually meant. Dad gave me a gift — a gift to look and see that I have an unknown depth of information available about me, inside. He recognized and taught me all those years ago that our thoughts and perceptions of ourselves and the world we live in create our destiny, our reality and we get to choose how it gets played out. All we have to do is ask the questions and our internal awakening, our wisdom, shall deliver the answers.

I never went to Wimbledon. My coach arrived at training not long after that day and said he was moving to Germany to coach over there. That was the end of my training days; I've only picked up a racket perhaps three or four times since. The situation played out perfectly and was a true testament to the idea that the power of what you focus your mind on creates your reality. My mind created the scenario so I wouldn't have to play at Wimbledon — the fear of playing locked itself so powerfully into my mind that I created the situation for me not to play. I was so scared of the unknown I wanted to stay where I was familiar; in the place and with the people where I could predict what would happen on a daily basis. To fly halfway around the world at the tender age of 13 to a country I knew little about to play in one of the most prestigious tournaments felt too overwhelming.

When we are in a situation where the boundaries are being stretched and we are less than comfortable, we tend to retreat back to a familiar place, just like I did in the above example of my life. People are faced with this every day when dis-ease or disease enters into the body. The signs and symptoms make people uncomfortable and in so doing they retreat back to known levels of comfort. This is where the mechanistic model of health care caters to the majority of the population. Comfort can be sought instantaneously.

There are three "circles" we journey between in the search for the understanding of the world and how it relates to us, others and our environment.

Firstly there is the "known" — what we know to be real or unreal — our history; what we consciously and unconsciously know [Diagram 9A]. We generally feel comfortable in this circle because we can predict to a degree what will happen. There is familiarity in our lives: people, places, events, times, things and so forth. We are comfortable here — this circle is about the application of our knowledge on a daily basis. It enables us to gather facts and create an abundance of knowledge which we define as our intellect. This is the place where we retreat back to when our world is challenged.

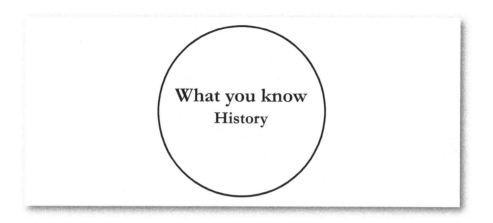

Diagram 9A: What you know

The next circle is the area of "what you know that you don't know" [Diagram 9B] or rather the "mystery" of life and the universe. Often we are happy to explore this new realm, knowing that we can retreat back into the familiar when too challenged. This is the area where our intuition is explored and followed.

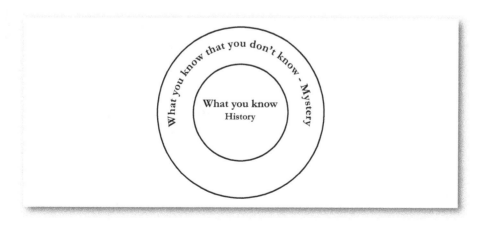

Diagram 9B: What you know that you don't know

When the mystery of "what you know that you don't know" gets incomprehensible and our boundaries are stretched, we retreat back into a state of knowing and surround ourselves once again with familiar people, places, events, times, and things. This second circle is where growth occurs. As we gain new information, the boundaries of what we know — our history — enlarges to encompass new understandings and new attempts. The beauty of this is that as we take the plunge towards the boundaries, from the "known" towards this "unknown", our knowledge of ourselves and the universe enlarges. Our mystery slowly starts to become our history, and so the cycle continues. We are continuously searching for new ways to enlarge the history circle. This is intuitive growth. Growth occurs when we have a balanced perspective of a given situation. We are able to see both sides: the positive and negative; the support and the challenge. When we have a situation where there are balanced, inspirational moments coinciding with love and gratitude, growth takes place and our mystery becomes our history. These moments enable certainty and presence.

The last circle is the notion of "you don't even know that you don't know". Here we don't even know how to ask the right questions. Imagine searching for the understanding of life by searching in an area you don't even know that you don't know anything about.

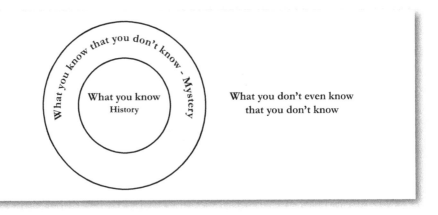

Diagram 9C: What you don't even know that you don't know

As our knowledge in history and mystery become enlarged, so too does the unknown. When we gain knowledge we also gain the realization of how little we really know. So the circle perpetuates. The idea that "you don't even know that you don't know" is constantly present in our search for greater understanding. Socrates was so right when he wrote *"I am the wisest man alive, for I know one thing, and that is that I know nothing."* I now look on my possibility to venture to England at the tender age of 13 with new eyes.

Everything we experience builds direction and purpose into our lives.

When I was 19 years old I was selected into the Australian Rowing team. It was a huge day for my ego and me. One of the National selectors rang me at home in Melbourne and said I had been selected into the National team and asked whether I could get to the Institute of Sport in Canberra by the following Thursday. I said absolutely! Running downstairs, I screamed the news to Mum and then rang Dad at work. It was a Thursday — I had a week in which to shout it from the rooftop and say goodbye to family and friends.

Upon my arrival in Canberra I felt so alone. People at the Institute of Sport rarely looked at you and they certainly didn't speak very often. Everybody was so focused. So that's what I became — extremely focused on the job at hand and winning, winning, winning. I wanted the Olympics and the gold medal. My boundaries were pushed on a daily basis. Was I stepping out into the mystery? Yes. Was I on my own and working out the unknown for myself? Yes.

I traveled overseas with the team and found this liberating. Our first overseas trip was to Seattle in Washington State, USA. I found myself outside of my comfort zone in the area of mystery but there was something so exciting about being in that zone. The team was billeted out to various families for a few nights which was a new experience, too. Almost twenty years on, I still keep in touch with the family who accommodated me.

After almost ten years in the sport and traveling overseas a number of times as well as back and forth from the Institute, I decided I had some questions to ask myself. I was operating at such a high intensity and starting to enjoy it less. Perhaps it was time to pursue other things. I was in two minds, as I wanted to attend the Olympics, but in that particular year it was decided not to send women. Apparently we weren't going fast enough, despite the times in training. I decided I didn't want to hang around for another four years to be told the same thing. I remember going home one weekend and lying on my bed. My Dad noticed that I was not in the best of moods, that I had something on my mind. I was on the verge of tears when he came into my room. The big question had come out of my mouth: I asked him if I should retire, take a break or do something else. Dad's response was, "Well, ask yourself and you shall have the answer. Only you know the answer to the question."

I wasn't too sure what I would do if I retired from rowing. I just knew I loved sport and teaching. Then one day at the Institute of Sport I was checking my mailbox and found a letter from a Physical Education College. I double-blinked and thought, "Isn't this a coincidence! I'm looking at retiring and wondering what to do next and bingo — a letter arrives in the mail and tells me what I'll be doing." It was a letter asking me to apply to the College — I couldn't believe it. I rang Dad and Mum, so excited. I was torn between the thought of retiring from rowing and pursuing other avenues. I decided there and then that I wanted to find out who I was when I didn't have sport in my life.

A disagreement with the rowing Head Coach saw me retire at the perfect time. I'd been focusing on where I wished to move on to after rowing and the disagreement enabled me to act on what was being presented. Within two days, I was back at home awaiting my acceptance into Physical Education College. Thanks to Dad and all his wisdom — he's a man who rarely judges or answers my questions. He knows that I have the answers; I just have to ask the questions. Taking myself out into the mystery of my life enabled me to move on from where I was at the time. My ability to focus and the trust I had in asking myself the next question of what I wanted to do in my life enabled me to further extend my history and mystery circle which allowed other avenues to open up.

The 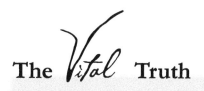 Truth

- Acknowledging that we are a part of a greater universe can sometimes seem overwhelming to accept. We retreat to a world where we have knowing and certainty — we seek comfort in the predictable outcome of certain people, places, events, times, and things.

- Next time you are presented with the possibility of having your reality expanded, stop and take note of where you are and in what frame of mind you are viewing this new information. It just might very well be the information you require there and then to make a leap into the unknown and expand your boundary.

The Vital Questions

- Write about a situation in which you felt your boundaries had been challenged and staying in your history was more comforting than venturing forth into the mystery, the unknown.

- Write about a time where your lights were turned on, a time when you embraced the mystery and you found it hard, as a result, to view your life in the same way?

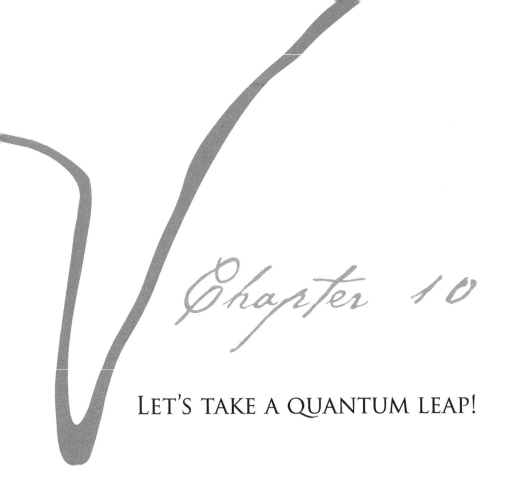

Chapter 10

LET'S TAKE A QUANTUM LEAP!

"How wonderful that we have met with a paradox. Now
we have some hope of making progress."[5]

NIELS BOHR,
1922 NOBEL PRIZE IN PHYSICS

It is interesting that the information available today suggests that our thoughts create our reality. If you'd like to research proponents of this theory, look up Dr. Deepak Chopra M.D., Dr. Demartini, D.C., Dr. Bruce Lipton, Ph.D., Dr. Wayne Dyer, Ph.D., and Dr. B.J. Palmer, D.C. People are even making docu-dramas about this school of thought today. I believe this concept to be true, and it's something I was taught during my college education. If our thoughts create our reality, how then can we change our thoughts to create the reality we want to manifest? How can we create the spiritual, mental, vocational, familial, financial, social and physical benefits in our world? What do we require in order to do this?

The first is to get to a state of balance. This is the state of internal equilibration where everything inside is working harmoniously together. The pathways of neurological communication are free of interference in this state of being. Our bodies are thus more able to adapt internally to the ever-changing outside world. States of gratefulness and love are more readily available upon equilibration of the system. When we reach a state where we are grateful for all the perceived positive and perceived negatives in our lives, we are at "zero point": where everything is connected to everything else via energetic forms. I believe that in this place lies the answer to life itself.

Zero point is timeless, mass-less and space-less. At this point you can create your future and even impact the past. Quantum mechanics tell us that you can exist in more than one place at a time. It tells us you live in the midst of limitless possibilities. These possibilities surround us and it is not until you choose to collapse onto one of these possibilities that the situation is able to become observable.

So you see there are many possibilities and potentials for a given situation. Here's the key…we get to CHOOSE the outcome. We get to CHOOSE what we collapse on. We get to CHOOSE. Anything we can think about is possible to create. If we think it, it can happen. The probability that something can be created is based on the knowledge and focus we as the observers and choice makers give to the situation.

Each person is a reality maker. In forming our own reality it is important to make sure we as the observers are viewing both sides: the positive and negative, the support and challenge, the benefits and the drawbacks. When viewed in this light we are then able to clearly see the reality of the situation. We are creating our reality according to our observations of the world in which we live. Each person chooses which waves of consciousness and energy they will collapse into particles of experience called reality. This is why many people have different experiences of a situation which at first glance appears straightforward. We live in our own world, creating our own experiences and choosing our own outcomes according to what we choose to see as our reality. We do this in all seven areas of life: spiritual, mental, vocational, financial, familial, social and physical.

So how does all this relate to health? You get to choose. We create the states we wish to experience. The body has an amazing way of humbling us when we get too cocky, self righteous or egotistical. It brings us back to the state of internal and universal balance. Likewise, the body has a way of lifting us up when we drop ourselves too low. These are all states of reality where our thoughts are creating our state of being.

Julie, a middle aged lady, sought chiropractic care for the first time. Upon going through her history with her and asking her some questions to find out her primary reason for coming in for care, she shared her story about her hypothyroidism for which she had been on medication for seven years. After helping her body structurally stabilize we thought it would be a good idea to work on the emotional and chemical component of her wellbeing. In this way she was able to see where she was stuck in her life and why she was manifesting this perceived state of illness in her body. There was some perceived benefit to what she was experiencing and why she was manifesting it further. Julie was only seeing one side, the drawbacks, and ignoring the benefits.

IN FORMING OUR OWN REALITY IT IS IMPORTANT TO MAKE SURE WE AS THE OBSERVERS ARE VIEWING BOTH SIDES: THE POSITIVE AND NEGATIVE...

Julie had been through a divorce some nine years prior and was married two years later. Remembering that Julie had manifested hypothyroidism some seven years ago — around the time of the re-marriage — I asked her about her relationship and she replied that it was "all right." Julie never gave too much away, but it wasn't difficult to read her like a book. The weaker of the two in the relationship, all she wanted was to be happy. Julie was constantly telling herself she was happy. That's what she wanted to believe, however, her perceived hypothyroidism was telling her otherwise. Julie hadn't yet awakened herself to the internal message her hypothyroidism was giving her.

Happiness is an illusion. In its gift to the world, quantum mechanics tells us that there are two sides to everything. We hear ourselves saying it too, don't we? We hear people saying, "Well, I'll wait to hear the other side", "there are two sides to the story" and so forth. Thoughts are energy and energy has two polar sides: a positive and a negative. One cannot have happiness without sadness, success without failure, war without peace, dark without light and certainly not health without disease. We are forever changing according to our perceptions of our reality.

After a series of regular adjustments, Julie soon started to see where and why she was creating the state of dis-ease in her body. She could now see the benefits rather than just the drawbacks: one of which was more attention from her husband. Her husband was a cleaner and was out all night cleaning commercial properties so they rarely had time together in the evenings, and during the day he was sleeping. Julie felt like a single woman and yet she was married. She knew this about her husband prior to entering into the marriage, however when in the day-to-day routine of the relationship she obviously found it hard to cope with. When she came to this realization of gaining greater attention from her husband, she was freed, liberated. After a period of time, Julie found herself stopping the thyroid medication and making changes in the home environment that were more supportive of where she was at and what she valued. It was only a few months later that she had the internal understanding and felt safe and powerful to step out into the world on her own again. In doing so, Julie acknowledged her desire to move on and so separated and later divorced her husband. When Julie was in the relationship, she was living up to somebody else's perceived understanding of the world and not being true to what she really wanted in her life. She had been in a relationship where she felt she had to create states of disease and dis-harmony in order to get what she wanted. After finding out through the adjustments and conversations we had that she wasn't living according to what she wanted and what was most important to her, she finally took responsibility for what she was creating and was able to turn it around.

This is not an uncommon situation that I have seen in practice. Nobody can have you live according to what they want. Live for what you want and I am sure you'll live a lot longer.

At the age of four I was watching a news segment on TV. It was a conference set-up and out walked a doctor of medicine with his surgery clothes, hat and mask dangling around his neck. He sat behind the microphones and told of the surgery he had just performed. It was the first of its kind in brain surgery. I was mesmerized by this surgeon and found him to be all over the TV that night and the papers the next day. I thought him a genius to be able to open up somebody's brain and perform surgery on it and have the person still alive the following day. From that day forth I wanted to be a brain surgeon, a doctor who would help change people's lives too. I would think about it all the time and to this day hold the picture of the TV interview clearly in my mind.

There was one thing stopping me from obtaining my dream when I started school. I was told by many a teacher that I wasn't very smart, (certainly not smart enough to be a doctor of medicine and surgery) nor was I any good at reading and writing, let alone comprehension. I was constantly challenged with spelling tests and examinations of any kind. I did have one area of specialty — sport. Acquaintances and teachers would tell my parents that I was brilliant at all sports and all I needed to do was specialize and I would have a successful career. I wasn't too keen on being a successful sports person, although at times I entertained the idea — all I wanted to be was a doctor.

In Grade Six I was attending a wealthy private school in Melbourne, Australia. When it was time for English class I would get a knot in the pit of my stomach, my head would bow down, and I would dread the words that came from my teacher's mouth: "Sarah, it's time for you to go to Miss Claire." Everybody knew who Miss Claire was. Oh, those words packed such a punch for me. When I already felt challenged with my English, it was a low blow to be called out in front of the class and have it announced that I was going to remedial English. As I walked out the door fellow students would stare and say, "Have fun!"

I HELD A VISION TO BE A DOCTOR AND CHANGE PEOPLE'S LIVES

As I exited the classroom door I would turn right and walk across a pebble-stoned pathway and out along a vast grassed area. The little brown door of Miss Claire's was just on the other side of the small oval. Every day, twice a day (there and back) as I crossed the small oval on my way to Miss Claire's office, I would say to myself, *"I will be a doctor and change people's lives."*

I held a vision to be a doctor and show all the people in the classroom that I *was* intelligent. In the class's presence I felt so inferior. I didn't know there were different types of doctors; I just wanted to be a brain surgeon. After completing a degree in physical education, a graduate diploma in psychology and a degree in general science, I received my wish of becoming a doctor.

And so here I sit, some 36 years on from the young four-year-old who held a vision of being a brain surgeon. I held this vision for some 20 odd years. Today I am a Doctor of Chiropractic, and every day I get to affect people's central (brain and spinal cord) and peripheral (everything outside of the brain and spinal cord) nervous systems. I get to help people change their lives.

Our thoughts truly do create our reality. We have the power to create what it is that we want in our lives.

The *Vital* Truth

- We choose our reality, in all seven areas of life.

- In any of the seven areas of life in which we are in a state of balance and equilibration, we collapse the situation we require in order to provide what it is we wish to manifest in our lives.

- Quantum Mechanics enables people to explore the polar opposites of a situation: the negative and the positive, the support for and the challenge against.

The *Vital* Questions

- What do you want to create for yourself?

- Picture a warehouse with a roller door on the front. Slowly roll up the door. Inside are all the experiences you wish to have in this lifetime (people, places, things, ideas, events etc). Write what you see behind the door. If you can see them, you can create them.

Your notes

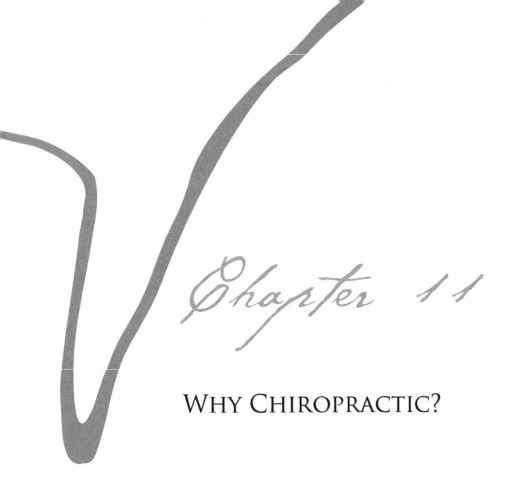

Chapter 11

WHY CHIROPRACTIC?

"The doctor of the future will give no medicine but will interest his patients in the care of the human frame, in diet and in the cause and prevention of disease."

THOMAS EDISON (1847-1931)

The time was the 1800s. The industrial revolution was well underway. Factories were ablaze with smoking chimney stacks and people were certainly optimistic about their futures. In Davenport, Iowa, a little town on the Mississippi, boats were delivering cargo and picking up material to take elsewhere. In this bustling town a discovery was about to emerge, a discovery that would change the direction of health care in the immediate present and foreseeable future. A discovery so great that people's lives would change as a result. Some would embrace and integrate this new understanding whilst others would be challenged and threatened and as a result try to stop the spread of this vital truth.

A young gentleman by the name of Daniel David Palmer (later to become known as "D.D.") had an office in the Ryan building in downtown Davenport. He was working as a magnetic healer at the time and was about to discover one of the world's best-kept secrets. The building's janitor told D.D. that he had been deaf for 17 years and when D.D. offered to check the young janitor, he found a displaced vertebra. D.D. offered to adjust the displaced vertebra and with Harvey Lilliard's permission he set about doing just that. After the adjustment, Harvey Lilliard said to D.D. that he could hear once again the sound of the horse and cart over the cobbled roads. Within a week Harvey had his hearing restored. Although the act of replacing displaced vertebra into their proper position had been practiced across the globe for hundreds and hundreds of years, it was D.D. Palmer who was the first person to write about the connection between the nervous system interference and the functioning of the body.

Chiropractors are taught that the nerve system is the master system of the body. It innervates all the cells, tissues, organs and systems. This philosophy has not changed today.

The vitalistic (chiropractic) and the mechanistic (medicinal) models of health became more prominent in the 1800s and these two became the dominating health care professions. Interestingly both of these professions have ties to Hippocrates, the Greek physician. It was Robert Koch in 1860 who proposed the germ theory (yes — it is just a theory) and this was where modern Newtonianbased medicine and science as we know it today has decided to stay. It was in 1895 when Chiropractic arrived on the health scene with a very different message.

D.D. Palmer founded the idea of specific spinal adjustments introduced to the body in order to create optimum states of health. In the beginning Chiropractic wasn't about "treating" back pain for which it has now become known, much to the detriment of the profession and what its possibilities are. D.D. Palmer, said "Chiropractic was founded on tone...the sole purpose of Chiropractic is to reunite physical man with spiritual man."

Chiropractic has always been about connecting and reconnecting the individual (physical man) to the innate wisdom within (spiritual man) that exists within every living thing. When that connection and reconnection occurs, any and all things are possible. Your perception of your world and of the world that is around you will change. Most importantly, however, evolution is possible.

I remember when I was studying physical education at college, I thought I knew all about the body and, granted, I knew more than some people. I thought I knew how the body worked. I thought it was all based on the muscular system. How misinformed I was. It wasn't until I set myself up as a personal trainer and had such clients as NBL basketball players, Australian Touch Football players and the World Aerobic champions, that I first had my exposure to another form of health care.

CHIROPRACTIC HAS ALWAYS BEEN ABOUT CONNECTING AND RECONNECTING THE INDIVIDUAL (PHYSICAL MAN) TO THE INNATE WISDOM WITHIN (SPIRITUAL MAN)...

At first I felt rather threatened and intimidated. These people were doctors, but somehow I thought they didn't know what they were talking about. I certainly didn't think the body needed to be adjusted. My philosophy at the time was the complete opposite of where I find myself today and this is what I have found to be the difference: people who choose the mechanistic route became passive participants in their ability to express health. The doctor is the active participant and has the answers, the knowledge and the control over the patient. The passive participant is told germs create disease and as such are to be gotten rid of, destroyed. Vaccines were introduced to conquer all microbes and supposedly "protect" the victim, the passive participant. The mechanistic model educates people to rely on others for "health" which in turn creates an understanding that their own bodies don't know how to heal themselves.

Today we are still attracted to the idea that we must "get rid of something", "fix it", have instantaneous gratification and relief. We spend more money on our cars, gymnasium memberships and vacations then we do on our health.

Did you know the most money a government or insurance company spends on us is spent in the last 18 to six months of our lives? Why? Because they chase the symptoms for us. We are having surgery, x-rays, MRIs, CTs drugs, drugs and more drugs in order to "get rid of" whatever is happening in our bodies. We follow this route because we assume and have been taught to trust that the educated mind knows more than the intelligence of the body — hence the passive participant syndrome. Sadly enough, at this stage most of us aren't even aware of the implications to the body; we just want to be symptom-free. Interestingly, when we are symptom free we think we have our health back. Why is this, when the definition of health (see Chapter 5) states nothing about being symptom-free and having no pain? Why has society adopted the Health definition as that of "no pain"?

Health does not come from the outside in. It is only when people, who think within this model, get a symptomatic expression within their body that creates disharmony that they decide to do something about it at all costs. Prevention kicks in the day *after* we have a symptom in our body. I propose the question to you: wouldn't an optimum state of health be a more productive paradigm to live in, rather than residing in a paradigm that says "Do nothing, but when something happens fix it"?

People who seek the chiropractic philosophical understanding for their health care, on the other hand, find a very different message. They find a philosophy, which is a way of life. They are educated in the art, science and philosophy that their body has everything within it to express health to an optimum level. If symptoms are present, it is because there is interference to their nerve system. Interference creates imbalances within the body and ultimately changes how the body functions on a day-to-day basis.

D.D. Palmer said, "The chiropractor looks upon the body as more than a machine; a union of consciousness and unconsciousness; Innate's ability to transfer impulses to all parts of the body — the coordination of sensation and volition: a personified immaterial spirit and body linked together by the soul — a life directed by intelligence uniting the immaterial with the material."[6]

The 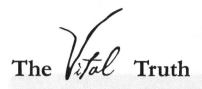 Truth

- There comes a time in a person's life when they begin to question what is real and unreal. For children this starts at the age of seven. Have you noticed in your own child or the children around you how they question, question, and question some more? They are searching for the truth in their reality.

- As an adult, it's time to question the information delivered to you.

The 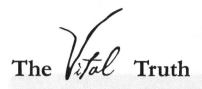 Questions

- Are you afraid to ask the questions and are you afraid to hear the answers? If you ask, you will be well-equipped to make a decision.

- Why would an optimum state of wellness be a more productive paradigm to live in than a "fix it" paradigm?

- What is your definition of health?

- What imbalances have you created in your life which have led to symptomatic expression?

- What awakening did the symptomatic expression give you?

- How did you integrate the experience into your life? Was it via mechanistic or vitalistic methods?

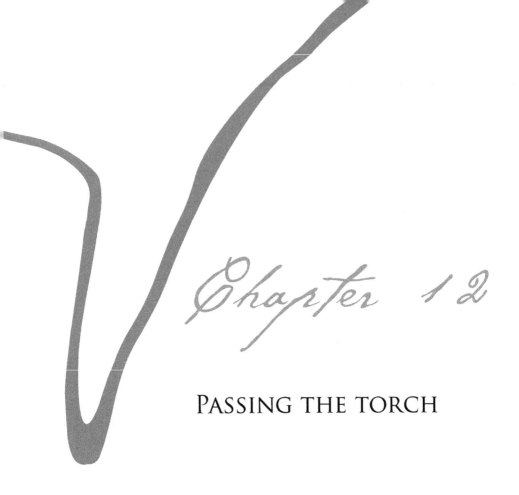

Chapter 12

PASSING THE TORCH

"You never know how far reaching something you think,
say or do will affect the lives of millions tomorrow"

B.J. PALMER

Bartlett Joshua (B.J.) Palmer, the son of Daniel David (D.D.) Palmer and known within the profession as the developer of Chiropractic, did much within and outside of the chiropractic profession to claim a rightful stake in the health care realm. D.D. passed the torch to B.J. and B.J. passed the torch to his son, David Daniel, known as the educator of Chiropractic. B.J., in my opinion, was one of the great philosophers of the last century. He was an eclectic gentleman who spoke his mind on many occasions to any and all who would listen. He loved travel and did much to spread the understanding of chiropractic philosophy around the globe. He acquired the second largest osteology collection in the world, which has now been bequeathed to Palmer College of Chiropractic.

When I chose to become a chiropractor a number of events took place that have enabled me to get to where I am today. This is a journey which demonstrates to you that when you're on your life's path everything just falls into place and life seems to be so easy.

It was a week night and we were heading out to dinner with our chiropractors who are also our friends. It was a going-away dinner for them because they were moving from Melbourne to Tasmania in the next few weeks. They had asked two other couples for dinner that night who we were yet to meet. There was something about this dinner that I was looking forward to, besides the beautiful place we were going to eat at. As we all sat around and shared stories, for some reason I felt compelled to ask them if they had the chance to study Chiropractic again, where would they go? They responded: Palmer College of Chiropractic.

"Where's that?" I asked.

"Davenport, Iowa," replied Benjamin. When asked why they would make that choice, both replied, "It's because of the philosophy." Pressed further, they pointed out that it is the founding school of the chiropractic profession, also referred to as the "Fountain Head"; it's "where it all began" well over a century ago.

The next day I found myself looking up Palmer College of Chiropractic on the Internet. It was about the time when the Internet was really getting up and running and Palmer College was redesigning their website. I managed to download a lot of information — I was in my final year of psychology at the time while working as the Victorian and Tasmanian personnel manager for Australia's largest international travel company. Wondering what I would do with my psychology knowledge, I read the information during a lecture break and was so overwhelmed that I was brought to tears. This was what I was looking for.

I went home that afternoon and told my husband that I was moving to America. You can imagine the look I received and the reply was a very long *"Okay…"* I would have left the next day — that's how sure I was of the commitment and move. I had no idea about how we would pay for it; I just knew I had to be there.

On a side-story, only three years prior I had sat on a park bench with my husband, in Vancouver's Stanley Park. We were enjoying the city lights at night, and I asked him if he thought we would ever study in the USA or Canada. He said he thought we would at some stage in our life. I shared with him that night what I used to visualize about as a young girl going through school.

"What was that?" he asked.

"Well," I said, "When I was at school a small group of us used to sit around and share visions of what we wanted to be and where we wanted to be in the future. Many of the girls said married by 22 perhaps and with a couple of kids by 24, driving the nice car and having a huge house. I never shared with them what I wanted I just had the knack of listening and nodding and not being asked. Inside, however, when they were sharing their stories with the group, I was sharing mine with myself. I always thought I

> I WENT HOME THAT AFTERNOON AND TOLD MY HUSBAND THAT I WAS MOVING TO AMERICA.

would marry an American." I wasn't too sure where it was coming from — I had just always had that vision. To my surprise, when my husband and I met, he shared with me he is an American citizen.

When I told my husband I was moving and he said a really dragged out *"okay"* he also added "I am going to have to think about this." And think he did. He thought long and hard about it for *three month*s. He decided that it was something he wanted to do also and so we both decided to make the move and study together.

Prior to our departure, I rang my brother-in-law to ask if he could ask his Dad when he went to bed that night if we were meant to go to America to study. My husband's father had passed away in 1993, and as a result his brother had become extremely psychic, often having conversations with his father. He called back the next morning.

"This is what Dad said — have you got a pen? — you are to go to America: it's extremely positive. You will find a place on top of a hill where all your illusions will be broken."

So with that, we set about organizing for things to be sent across to the States. Here I was, envisioning marrying an American, and it happened, and now I was seeing my vision fulfilled of studying in the States and becoming a chiropractor, a doctor that would inspire people to change their lives, to ask different questions.

We both went to see our psychic before we departed and she said three things that were the same to both of us: We will live overseas for a period of time and shall own a house there. With that, I saw the house that we then bought in the town. She said that there would be a tall man with dark hair who would be extremely positive in our time there. There was also to be a financial benefit, and she saw a group of eight other people all sitting around a table, discussing the future of something — she wasn't sure what.

There *was* a tall man there. He was the president of the College and a gentleman who was exceptionally nurturing to both my husband and I.

When we got to the fourth trimester we both were awarded the Vogt Leadership Scholarship — the award I mentioned in Chapter four. Only ten of these are given out at a time. We used to sit around at our meetings with eight other students discussing the future of Chiropractic.

What brought me to tears one day was the vision my brother-in-law had shared with us which his Dad had spoken of. When we arrived in the States, Iowa in particular, we thought, *Not too sure where this hill is that Dad was talking about!* Iowa is as flat as a tack. When we were halfway through our first trimester I was walking across the skywalk, a corridor which connects two of the buildings and has glass on either side, I turned to my husband and, grabbing his arm, led him over to the window.

"Do you see where we are?"

Plain as day, he replied, "We're in Iowa and I'm looking at the Mississippi River!"

"But *really* look where we are!"

He looked at me with a confused look on his face.

I yelled, "We're at the top of the hill!" This was the only hill in town. B.J. Palmer used to refer to "life on Brady Street Hill"! "This is the place where our illusions shall be broken!" I said. It had already started to happen.

From that day forth I have searched for the greater understanding of the chiropractic philosophy. It is my vision now to educate and enable other people to see the illusions that they may carry and pass on regarding health and life. I wish to share with billions of people the understanding of vitalistic philosophy and how it relates to health whilst encouraging people to study one of the most amazing professions available today. I wish to pass the torch to others in the desire to help them see new ways of being and gaining health. Who are you passing your torch to?

The 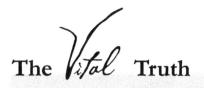 Truth

- The vitalistic philosophy of health and understanding is pure.

- Share this with your support network and people you want to challenge!

- Pass the torch.

The *Vital* Questions

- Have you thought about studying Chiropractic?

- If you had one idea to share with the world, what would it be?

- Do you have an inspiration for which you would like to "pass a torch"?

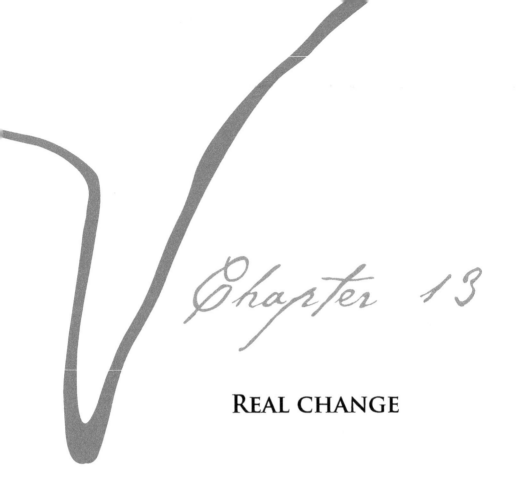

Chapter 13

REAL CHANGE

"Correct skeletal alignment is essential for a healthy body, mind and spirit."

D.D. PALMER

When most people come into the practice, they are coming in "for" something and are carrying with them a particular symptom which they want rectified instantly. They have usually tried everything else: pills, herbal mixtures, a new exercise, fads and other health care professionals. Most have found one or a combination of them didn't deliver what "it" promised, or rather what they were expecting, which is usually instantaneous relief. We are constantly in search of one thing that will make us better, more stable or which will ultimately take the pain and/or discomfort away. We generally want the pleasure without the pain. However, the universal intelligence doesn't deliver one-sided emotions. Pleasure and pain are inversely proportional to one another. The innate intelligence of the body, however, is constantly searching for the balance point where there is a harmony between, for example, the pleasure and pain experience. There is no world in which exists only pleasure, just as there is nice and mean, good and bad, and so forth. We have all emotions within us. To expect one without the other is to set ourselves up for a fall in the equal and opposite direction.

"No doctor can heal, nor can anyone else produce healings for you, but when correct adjustments are made, the body's self-healing process begins and dis-ease turns to ease."

D.D. PALMER

There are no "outside-in" approaches in Chiropractic. Chiropractors work with our internal knowing and understanding to allow the body to reach new states of being. The skull and spinal column house the most precious piece of machinery ever designed: the central nerve system. This allows us to have a plethora of physical, chemical and emotional changes take place independently or all at the same time. How ingenious! Let me give you a special example of the difference chiropractic made in Caleb's life and that of his parents when his parents began to trust the body's innate intelligence:

Caleb was two years old when his mother brought him into the practice. Caleb had had a severe fall, which his mother didn't see, but she had noticed his left temporal area was red and a little swollen. A week after the fall, Caleb developed a hematoma in the brain and had started having seizures. His mother took him to their local medical doctor who self-assuredly told the mother that the fall had nothing to do with the seizures and that he had just developed epilepsy. Caleb's mother remained unconvinced, but left the doctor's suite with medication prescribed to control her son's epileptic seizures and to prevent him from having grand mal seizures.

Caleb's mother went ahead and administered the medication she had received from their medical doctor. After a period of time she noticed other changes. The body is remarkable in how it still chooses to release pressure from the increased neural activity in someone who has epilepsy even when medication is administered to "control" the seizures. There still needs to be an outlet to release the pressure that is building internally. When the body gets masked in its ability to express health it finds another way to give you the message. This is exactly what happened in Caleb's example. He ended up having what are called "drop attacks", where he would suddenly fall and be unconscious for a few seconds. The family lived on a farm and through their concern they had him wear a crash helmet. His parents started to become very concerned when things weren't changing and he was continuing to have these "drop attacks" with increased frequency. They felt there had to be something else that could help him and the family.

WHEN THE BODY GETS MASKED IN ITS ABILITY TO EXPRESS HEALTH IT FINDS ANOTHER WAY TO GIVE YOU THE MESSAGE.

About six months after the initial incident, his parents sought out chiropractic care, driving for two hours to reach the practice. Upon his initial adjustment Caleb was found to have pelvic instability as a result of the blow to the temporal area of the head. Only his pelvis was balanced that day, but there was still a large amount of cranial work to be done on the child following the initial adjustment.

The family returned home that night. Caleb's parents anxiously phoned later that evening, saying he had had a grand mal seizure despite him still being on the medication. They were advised not to panic. It was explained that it is normal for the body to release stress in the system and that Caleb's body would calm down. The parents trusted the advice, and did everything to make Caleb's night comfortable. After that night Caleb never had a grand mal seizure again. His drop attacks went from 20 per day to only three or four each day. A few years later his drop attacks were reduced to one or two per week, and then eventually became almost non-existent.

Caleb's life was changed immensely through the care that was sought and his body's inborn ability to change. And it was not only his life, but the lives of his parents that have changed. New eyes were opened to the potential of the human body.

Your nervous system allows for vital accurate information to be communicated between your brain and body and back again. Where there is interference there is also a decrease in your body's ability to express health, whether it is physical, chemical or emotional.

An adjustment allows us to be the best we can be, to reach our full potential and function at our optimum level. There is no discrimination against sex, age, race, religion or species. If you have a nerve system, then it is important to get it checked.

The *Vital* Truth

- If you mask the communication in your body, it creates new ways in which to awaken you to what is occurring internally.

- Learn to listen to your body's messages and make the changes.

- Seek other understandings in health and vitality.

- Give yourself and your family the gift of regular adjustments.

The *Vital* Questions

- Will you incorporate chiropractic care into the life of you and your family?

- Do you know of a child and/or a parent who could benefit from regular care and a new-found understanding of how the body functions?

- Are you ready to explore options that may look as though they run contrary to popular medical opinion?

Your notes

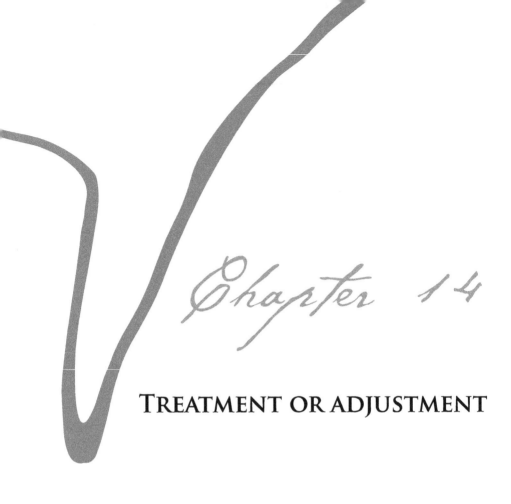

Chapter 14

TREATMENT OR ADJUSTMENT

"Insanity: doing the same thing over and over again and expecting different results."

ALBERT EINSTEIN (1879-1955)

I n looking at the philosophical underpinnings of the various health professions we have visited two vastly different understandings of gaining health. On the one side we see the "outside- in" approach to health (mechanistic, medicinal, treatment) and on the other side we see an "inside-out" approach to health (vitalistic, chiropractic, adjustment). In order to understand them that little bit better and see the differences between them, let's take a closer look at what each one does.

Firstly let's take a look at the term *treatment.* To treat something implies that the participant is passive in the whole process of health. *Dorland's Pocket Medical Dictionary* states that treatment is "management and care of a patient or the combating of disease or disorder."[7] This suggests health is something that you gain and lose and then is given back to you by somebody other than yourself. It also implies that disease is something that should be fought, gotten rid of, which is a disempowering approach, to say the least. Why would people want to eradicate the symptoms and signs which communicate to us that something is occurring in the body? Even the 1901 Nobel Prize winner Emil von Behring (considered the founder of the science of immunology) thought disease should be combated and eradicated, leading him to spend his life in pursuit of developing vaccines, all in the name of *treating* something and someone.

However, there are many different ways to look at the advent of disease, dis-ease, and symptomatic expressions in the body. Further, there are many areas within our lives which can coerce the body into symptomatic expression: thoughts (emotional), trauma (physical) and toxins (chemical) as outlined in Chapter four.

So what are adjustments and how can they serve the body in growth? *The Macquarie Concise Dictionary* states an adjustment is "to bring into a satisfactory state; to adapt; to accommodate; to fit as one thing to another." Adjustments are specific, small lever introductions of forces into the body in order to create clear levels of communication within the nerve system, thereby re-establishing homeostasis (balance) within the body. Adjustments enable the body to adapt to an ever-changing internal and external environment.

When the nerve system is unable to clearly communicate with itself (neurological interference), dis-ease sets into the body. This altered state of communication affects the messages between the cells, tissues, organs and systems, resulting in many different symptomatic expressions. Picture the old TV "rabbit ears" (set-top antenna), for a moment. Do you remember a time when your television went all fuzzy? What did you do? I imagine you stood up, walked over to the antennae and adjusted the rabbit ears ever so specifically and slightly in a purposeful direction in order to create better communication for the purpose of displaying a clearer picture? This is exactly what adjustments do within the body. They enable the nerve system to communicate with itself, allowing for clearer messages to be expressed.

Disease is a necessity for the body. Some people may stumble, cry and no doubt become outraged at the thought of this. This is because we have been indoctrinated into thinking otherwise for so long. Disease is *necessary* for the growth of our bodies, and symptomatic expression is but one part of that.

What happens to a child when they get a cold? Do you have them adjusted or do you treat what is present in their system? When I say a cold I don't just mean the expression of the cold in the rosy cheeks, cough, perhaps sinus congestion and dribble from the nose, but have you *really* noticed what is going on in their bodies? Their body, just like an adult's, works at its optimum capacity to make sure that the entity in the body is contained within the ring of fire. The ring of fire is one of our first lines of defense, and it just so happens that this is where the tonsils sit. Inflammation of the tonsils (tonsillitis) indicates immunity is being built. The tonsils are working to build immunity to the entity and there are many, many cells involved in this process. Imagine doing bicep curls all day. Would your muscles hypertrophy (enlarge) and would you let off a little heat and sweat and perhaps be tired at the end of it and need a little rest before you went at it again? Yes. It is no different for our tonsils. They are working hard to build all the chemical reactions required

DISEASE IS A NECESSITY FOR THE BODY. SOME PEOPLE MAY STUMBLE, CRY AND NO DOUBT BECOME OUTRAGED AT THE THOUGHT OF THIS.

to contain the entity in the ring of fire. Obviously a system that is free of nerve interference can do this at an effective, efficient and faster rate, whilst at the same time letting off a little heat to help burn the entity — much the same way as you might sterilize a bottle in boiling water. They then require some rest before they go at it again. It takes 7-14 days to build natural immunity. Has there been a time in your life where you have gone to your local doctor and he/she has said if it doesn't change in 7-14 days then come back? A body which can communicate with itself has an increased chance at building natural immunity faster.

What if the person doing the bicep curls were given an extra 20 pounds to lift? Would this cause concern? Would the focus be on the 20 extra pounds they now had to lift? This happens with the body when a drug is introduced. Its focus is now upon two entities: the drug and the bacterium/virus. So, building immunity becomes challenged as one is trying to build while the other is trying to suppress. Now add an encumbered nerve system and you have a system that is quite compromised.

The body is constantly working to reach new milestones. Foolhardy is the person who tries to stop this process — not only in infants and children, but adults too. Also foolhardy is the person who is proud of the fact that they never get "sick". They are missing an opportunity to grow. I was told by the late Dr. Fred Barge, D.C., a past lecturer at college, that a runny nose can be stopped in three days. He said to get some tissue and plug up your nose. The art of sneezing, he said, is innate, it's inborn and the rate at which we externally propel internal substances via the sneeze can exceed a speed of 100 mph (over 160km/hr)! Dr. Barge said children are taught to blow their nose, a process that is not innate to our wellbeing. When we blow our nose, we propel the internal substance at such slow speeds that the bacterium is propelled backwards into the nasal cavity and sinuses which perpetuates the cold further. Next time you have a runny nose, reach for the tissues and plug up the nose — it will be over before you know it.

With your children — well, anybody really — it is important to wait the 7-14 days that it takes to build natural immunity and just love them, hug them and support them with what is expressing through their bodies. If drugs are administered the body gets confused. The body now has to deal with a drug *and* the entity as we have already seen. Let's take a fever, for example: if you wait for the fever to break naturally and refrain from putting drugs into the body, then you will notice advancement. There will quite possibly be a change in eating, growth, dexterity, language, teeth, crawling, walking and so forth. Parents and primary care givers who choose to give children medication to soothe the symptomatic expression may wish to reconsider their view of health. In today's Western society, it seems that it takes courage by some parents and primary care givers to allow a child to go through the expression and reach new milestones as a result. Instead, parents or primary care givers usually look on the child with pity or with their own pain and judgment, through their own filtered glasses. What is necessary is a body that can communicate with itself. When it can do this there is no requirement for external remedies to take symptoms away — the body just takes care of it and at times it does so without symptomatic expression.

Diseases are gifts to the body which are making you and your life extraordinary. We personally don't have a thermometer in the house, a medicine cabinet or drugs of any kind. If our children are hot and clammy and the thought might be that they're having a health expression, then we adjust them regularly throughout the course of the day and night for the purpose of helping their bodies to communicate with themselves, thereby enabling a clear pathway for their own body to deal with the symptomatic expression. They, and we, acknowledge that a system that can communicate with itself has far greater opportunity to support what is happening internally and as a result take them (and us) to new levels of understanding in their capabilities.

We were in Fiji not so long ago for a ten day holiday. Prior to traveling we were in the midst of designing our house renovation to accommodate our youngest, Anais, whom was yet to be born and also making decisions about activities and events in our lives. When we arrived in Fiji we were all exhausted and quite literally collapsed, relaxing on the beach, by the pool, reading books and making full use of the nanny service for our two young boys. We were about four days into the holiday when I noticed lots of what looked like mosquito bites on the boys' heads, faces and arms and slightly on their chests. They also appeared very fatigued. I had a headache, sinus congestion, cough and a general malaise. The boys were itching somewhat but not all the time. My husband and I adjusted them daily and within two days the "mosquito bites" had disappeared. Two days later I got some

> A FEVER IS A SYMPTOM OF AN ILLNESS — YES, A SYMPTOM. IT IS SOMETHING THAT YOUR BODY HAS CREATED.

"mosquito bites" over my shoulders, scalp and some over my legs. They weren't too itchy but I noticed them. I too was getting adjusted daily. It occurred to me on our return from Fiji that we had all had the chicken pox. The boys' bodies did a remarkable job with building immunity, as did mine. When something occurs naturally in the body and you allow natural immunity to build internally then the length of time of the symptomatic expression, in my observation, is reduced. The advances in social interaction, independence, food choice, height, dexterity and language were all areas where the boys gained growth after the chicken pox. It is truly incredible where their bodies take them to after such an encounter.

I believe it is a right of passage for all people to have this. Just allow the innate intelligence of the body to work its wonder and leave the educated mind out of it, as it causes more damage. Fevers, dis-ease, diseases and other health expressions are sent to children (and adults) as a means to enable growth. They enable new levels of immunity to be reached, new levels of the mind and body to be created, and ultimately allow them to pop to new levels of expression in health. Something that may have been seen as a problem in the past can now be seen as an opportunity for them and yourself.

A doctor or parent who tries to bring down a fever, as the late Dr.Strang, D.C. said, is "like a fireman who tries to turn off the fire alarm rather than find the fire." A fever is a *symptom* of an illness — yes, a symptom. It is something that your body has created. Dr. Strang says "fever has been shown to increase levels of interferon, an antiviral substance produced by the body and also increases blood levels of copper and zinc." So with this in mind, do you think a fever is important? People have this fear that there shall be brain injury as a result of the high fever. If brain injury results it is usually because the compromise is in the brain itself or in the meninges; it is not usually a result of a high fever. Parents can be warned against rugging up the child, self or partner to keep them "warm", as this confuses the internal workings of the body and actually cools it down internally, which in turn delays the body's ability to burn off the entity. This is because the senses from the outside are sending messages saying that the body is warm. Instead, it's best to leave the person at room temperature or in their natural environment.

Would you rather receive an adjustment, or treat "something" from the outside-in which ultimately interferes with the innate wisdom of the body? Having a body that can communicate with itself is far more beneficial to the overall building of immunity.

The 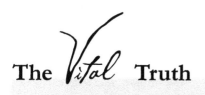 Truth

- Disease is *necessary* for the optimum growth of our bodies.

- Allowing the body to build natural immunity through overcoming disease brings advantages in all seven areas of life.

- It may take courage to allow symptomatic expressions; yet new understandings of the body's ability will be reached.

The *Vital* Questions

- What process do you go through when you or your child has a health expression?

- How do you think an unencumbered nerve system can help with healing?

- Knowing what you know now about the nerve system and the body's ingenious design, would you opt for treatment or regular adjustments?

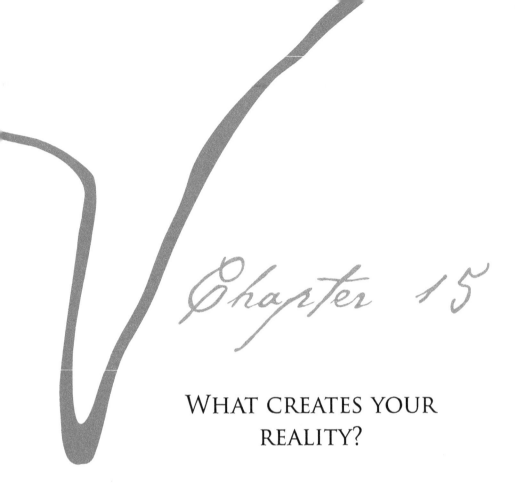

V

Chapter 15

WHAT CREATES YOUR REALITY?

"We are what we repeatedly do…."

ARISTOTLE

Many people come into the practice with a plethora of "things" happening within their body — lots of which they don't tell us about, regardless of how thorough we are in taking their history. One comment that does stand out to me is this notion of "genetics". I wish I had a dollar for every time a person has said to me, "My mother/father is a diabetic or is overweight or has heart disease," or one of many ailments. It's been my observation that people have been indoctrinated with the idea that they have no ability to change themselves. They see themselves as victims unto their bodies and their circumstances. People are constantly told they *are* their parents. The only ones who benefit are the pharmaceutical companies that have another avenue through which to sell their products. Companies constantly advertise "Take this to help reduce the symptoms of reflux, sinusitis, cough, heart disease …" Companies have even introduced vaccines to accommodate for the possibility of something occurring in your body, i.e. cervical cancer. "Let's get it before it becomes a problem" is often the unsung motto.

Knowing what you have read thus far about health, how to get it and where it comes from, can you see how ridiculous this sounds — putting something *into* the body to create health? How could that work? It is either ignorance or arrogance of the educated mind that would do such a thing to the innate intelligence and inner wisdom of the body. Whole communities these days are being checked to see if they have an ovarian cancer gene, the overweight gene, a diabetic gene, an intelligence gene and so forth. Why? For the benefit of business.

Genes are activated by perceptual signals sent by the brain to the cells, tissues and organs. This is the latest in the research of biological consciousness by Dr. Bruce Lipton.[8] Dr. Lipton, a renowned cell biologist, writes about the cell's hereditary units called chromosomes. In every cell nucleus there are 46 chromosomes, 23 from the mother's egg and 23 from the father's sperm. At the core of each chromosome is a long thread of DNA that represents the genes. Surrounding the DNA strand is a protein coat. The only way a gene can be expressed is if the protein coat is removed. This protein coat is removed via the interaction with environmental signals, many of which are provided through the nervous system in response to thoughts. If we truly believe the indoctrination that our genes rule us, we will create what we fear the most. *What we put our minds to creates our reality.* As Aristotle says, "We are what we repeatedly do…" These indoctrinated thoughts then enable a self-fulfilling prophecy to manifest. This sheds a whole new light on the nature/nurture debate.

Angela had been coming into the practice for some time. Her mother had recently passed away due to heart disease for which she had been on medication for a while. In her later years her mother was constantly in and out of hospital. On one particular office visit, Angela expressed her terror of "getting" the same condition as her mother and of dying young. She mentioned that over the preceding couple of days she had been having heart palpitations. After a series of questions, I asked Angela why she thought she was a victim to her own body. She found it difficult to answer the question. I explained to her that there isn't somebody out there waving a magic wand over her head saying, "I shall give you heart disease." Disease is not something that happens *to* us but something that we create *within* us. We are active participants in everything that we put out from ourselves and everything that we create within ourselves. We get to *choose* our state of being. We make the choices with the knowledge we have at the time. Angela found this information difficult to digest initially as the concept was so new to her. Angela soon realized, after a few more adjustments and some philosophical conversations, the impact the 3Ts have on our internal state of being. Angela and her family are still under care today as a result of the encounter we had over genetics. She got it. She realized she is the captain of her own ship, the creator of her own destiny.

DISEASE IS NOT SOMETHING THAT HAPPENS TO US BUT SOMETHING THAT WE CREATE WITHIN US.

Craig was brought in by his parents at two weeks old, having been referred by a local midwife. He was the first child for Mum and Dad who were in their late 30s and early 40s. There was lots of energy around how precious this little gift was. He was unable to fully latch onto the breast, having difficulty making a seal and not wanting to remove his tongue from the hard palate. He could not turn his head left at all and was already flattening on the right posterior occiput as a result.

After his first adjustment, Craig demonstrated an immediate change in sucking and began feeding regularly and with ease off the left breast. Mum and Dad calmed down phenomenally.

On the day of his fourth adjustment, Mum and Dad noticed his mood was calm on the day of the visit, however he was unsettled the day after, which they found confusing and of concern. An emotional technique was run which revealed him having low self esteem — being loved so much and not being "okay" to heal. As the parents became more aware of the situation, the energy dissipated and he became settled the day after an adjustment as well.

By the seventh adjustment, mild improvements in passive left rotation of the neck were observed, however he was still not turning naturally to the left. It was noted that his crying was now delayed; i.e. he would turn and then cry. It became obvious that it wasn't a physical distress, so another emotional technique was run on him, isolating that particular upper cervical area. It went back to not being okay to turn away from the right. Yet turning *to* the right was no problem. The emotional technique revealed there was a vanishing twin syndrome (when one of the fetuses in a twin pregnancy spontaneously aborts) on his left in-utero. Three days later, he turned his head to the left by himself for the first time. The parents were exceptionally grateful for the change he had made in his body in such a short space of time.

Craig continues to have regular adjustments. Mum and Dad are very aware of his environment and they have made gradual changes to other areas of his life such as diet, sleeping positions and routine as a result of the emotional techniques and the awareness they have gained through watching the changes in their son, and through the education provided to them about the body and how health is expressed.

Craig's parents grew to understand that the perceptions they had towards their precious son needed to be altered to allow him the freedom to heal. They were delighted with the changes brought about by the chiropractic care and were willing to love their child in a way that gave him room to grow.

Our perceptions towards ourselves and towards others are powerful. We are what we repeatedly do and what we repeatedly see. Craig's parents, through care, were able to see their contribution to his health expression and make the necessary changes in order to let him grow according to his own requirements and needs. It is important for us to evaluate how we see others to ensure we aren't restricting their growth through our own needs for them to be a certain way. Importantly, we need to check our perceptions of ourselves.

If we know that our perceptions create our reality, then we must also be aware that our thoughts shall determine our destiny. If we are focused on diabetes, heart disease, strokes, cancer, and so forth then we are likely to manifest these into our lives — it's the law of attraction. The genetic paradigm becomes a self-fulfilling prophecy to those who focus on it. The revelation is that *we are not our parents*. We are not victims. We get to choose how to do our lives. Our perceptions of our reality enable these choices to be executed.

The 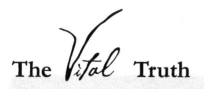*Vital* Truth

- Genetics is a *theory* based science.

- New research in this area is indeed showing us that our perceptions trigger an expression.

- Our world is viewed through our own perceptions.

- If a situation is focused on for long enough then it's created.

- We get to choose the way we want to live, how we want to live and what we bring into our lives.

- If we know we have the choice then we know we can make the required changes to liberate us to optimum levels of health expression.

The *Vital* Questions

- What perceptions and realities have you created around your own health and the health of others?

- Are you creating a diseased state in your body because of your thought processes and beliefs?

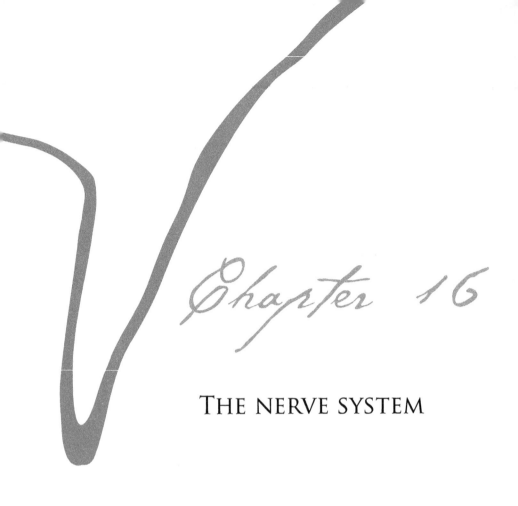

Chapter 16

THE NERVE SYSTEM

"…not a page, paragraph or even a sentence is found
in any one of the many works I have on anatomy,
neurology, physiology and pathology regarding the all
important fact that the position of bones has all to do
with the amount of nerve tension."

D.D. PALMER[9]

Let's take a look at the brain. The brain consists of three parts: the cerebral hemispheres, the cerebellum and the brain stem.

The cerebral hemispheres control higher functions such as our consciousness, attitude, beliefs and values, our knowing and our judgment. At this level we also have the ability to interpret and respond — the functional control of language and speech. Here we integrate all the incoming information so that we can respond to our environment in a normal manner. The cerebral hemispheres also control our ability to move voluntarily, enabling us to dress ourselves, move a foot to the brake peddle and so forth.

The cerebellum, or the hind brain, controls the functions of coordination, fine muscle movement, and balance.

The brain stem, or inner brain, houses all of the delicately balanced control centres that give you proper function. Some of these include respiration, digestion, and elimination. The nerves have their relay centres sitting in this part of the brain. Nature knows how to protect this delicate area, positioning the brain stem at the top of the neck, surrounded by the skull and vertebrae.

Dr. Vern Hagen, D.C. is a chiropractor in his 70s. He's been involved in the profession all his working life and still practices today. Over the course of his tenure in the profession he has been privy to many of the greats in all of the three primary areas of the profession: philosophy, science and art (technique). In one of his many lectures, he was sharing information about the brain stem. He said "the brain stem houses 90% of the nerve system. Take care of it and you take care of a lot of the neurological interferences in the body." It is in the brain stem area that the most delicate centres for control and coordination of all the cells, tissues, organs and systems of the body exist.

This area is of particular interest in the newborn baby. When a newborn baby arrives into the world via a vaginal birth or cesarean delivery, forceps, vacuum extraction and so forth, then neurological interference is of concern. Whatever the birthing method there is usually a degree of neurological interference that occurs.

When Zoe first came into the practice she was five days old. Sally, Zoe's mother had been told during the course of Zoe's birth that her baby was "stuck". Rather than allowing the body to move in posture and change in position, Sally was told to lie on the bed whilst the doctor pulled her baby out. Zoe's birth was by vacuum extraction. This was the firstborn for Sally and her husband, and not knowing what to expect, she had surrendered to the advice of the "medical" team. Upon Zoe's birth the nurse assigned to Sally noticed the feeding challenges and sleep disturbance on top of the obvious cranial distortions and thought that something else might be challenging Zoe. Our practice has a professional relationship with the local hospitals, midwives and nurses. We provide education for them in chiropractic philosophy and neurological interference and the impact this has on the developing body. Sally was told by one of the nurses in the hospital to go and see a chiropractor. Sally was perplexed at the thought of a chiropractor adjusting her newborn's bones, however was at a loss as to what to do. Sally thought it couldn't be any worse than what she was going through already. Zoe had a large cranial distortion as a result of the vacuum extraction — her parietal, occiput and temporal bones were distorted on her left side. Feeding was a challenge and sleepless nights were common. Sally was exhausted and her husband wasn't sure how to support the two of them.

During the initial consultation, Sally's mind was put to ease as to what a chiropractor does and it was explained to her what was going to happen. After Zoe's initial adjustment she slept soundly for the first time in five days. After two weeks of care Zoe's cranium had returned to a state of balance and the distortions were virtually unrecognizable. Sally was encouraged to continue breastfeeding. It was explained to her and her husband that the sucking motion helps to open up the cranium and aid the pumping of the cerebro-spinal fluid, the fluid that encases the brain and spinal cord. Sally and her husband's lives were changed as a result of the care they received for their young girl. They both continue to be advocates of the

AFTER ZOE'S INITIAL ADJUSTMENT SHE SLEPT SOUNDLY FOR THE FIRST TIME IN FIVE DAYS.

profession and have encouraged many a family to come in to receive care in the knowing that when all else seemed to fail, chiropractic and the vitalistic philosophy changed their lives and the life of their child.

It has been my observation in practice that when the nerve system is balanced, just like in little Zoe's situation, many of the symptomatic expressions people came into the practice with actually self-limit or go into self-remission.

If we take a closer look at the nerve system — the body's communication system — we notice a series of intricate and well-designed wires leading in many different directions. To the untrained eye it would seem chaotic, but the body knows what to do every time, one hundred percent of the time, provided there is no interference. There are thousands upon thousands of nerves, all of which come together at the base of the skull to form the spinal cord. There are thirty-three pairs of nerves coming from the cord itself and each branches and branches with other nerves in order to innervate all the cells, tissues, organs and systems of the body. This then creates one hundred percent coordinated function, which further enables the expression of health to take place. If we look closely at the cellular level we see twelve *different* nerve fibers innervating it. Remember, this is only at the cellular level. Furthermore, there is an average of 100,000 synaptic endings for every nerve fiber. There are, therefore, over 1.2 million nerve endings that are constantly hooking up in various intricate ways to innervate *one cell*. The body truly is ingenious in design and the more I learn about it the more I am humbled by the intelligence that runs it.

The spinal cord itself is an extremely delicate structure and therefore needs protection. The wisdom of the body decided to encase the most delicate structure of all in a moveable bony structure called the skull. This wisdom — the innate intelligence — didn't stop at encasing just the brain but also realized the cord and the initial part of the nerves needed protection, and so further developed the individual moveable bones (vertebra) of the spinal column.

Now that we know how intricate the system is, you probably have also figured out the importance of keeping the communication system free of interference so that proper functioning and expression of health can take place. Remember nature needs no help, just no interference.

The *Vital* Truth

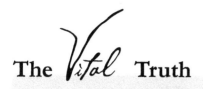

- The innate wisdom of the body houses the most delicate parts in two moveable bony structures called the skull and the spinal column.

- Chiropractors deal with the nerve system to enhance the body's ability to communicate with itself.

- When the nerve system is free of interference our capacity is limitless. We can truly do anything.

The *Vital* Questions

- Stand in front of the mirror and see where your eyes, ears, shoulders, hips, knees and ankles are in relation to each side. Is one side up and one side down? If you see the imbalances, perhaps it is time to get your body checked for neurological interference to increase your internal communication.

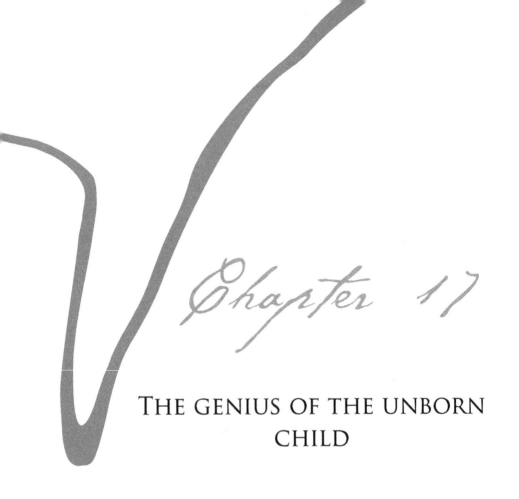

Chapter 17

THE GENIUS OF THE UNBORN CHILD

"Nature needs no help, just no interference."

B.J. PALMER

It's interesting to note that the power that made your body has the ability to heal your body. Imagine the difference if everybody in the world adopted this knowledge and lived by it — wouldn't the world's diseased conditions and illness rates be very different? No longer would we be putting synthetic formulas or tablets into the body thinking that this would improve health. It is most harmful to our longevity on this planet.

I have chosen to be part of a profession which has a philosophy that is a way of life; a philosophy that teaches that health is expressed from the inside out. Our ability to heal ourselves and express health is an innate knowing far greater than our educated minds. It also suggests we were born with a limitless potential to express health. Regaining, maintaining, growing, and educating ourselves in health is our responsibility. Based on our knowledge and understanding, we make choices for ourselves which in turn create our reality. What is important is to respect the life and intelligence within the body and know how amazing it is.

For the sheer purpose of increasing our awareness and out of respect for the internal intelligence that keeps us functioning every day of our life, let me illustrate the intricate order of events that take place in the design of making who we are as the physical being.

Upon ejaculation, the sperm knows what to do— not just once, but time and time again. They swim and swim and swim, competing against each other for the right to penetrate the ovum wall. Provided there is no interference, the sperm find their way to the egg every time. Upon fertilization there is now ALL the necessary cells to form a human being. Remarkable. Proteins, DNA codes, organs and nerves are ready to work harmoniously together to form a human being, and provided there is no interference this shall be complete at the end of nine months.

After three weeks, the intricacies of the construction call for an overseeing system to govern the ongoing development. It is at this stage that we see the formation of the brain and the nerve system to help coordinate this development and shall do so for the rest of our lives, provided there is no interference. The nerve system controls all the functions of the cells, tissues, organs and systems of the body within the embryonic stage through to the adult stage in the physical lifetime. The nerve system is responsible for the homeostasis mechanism which enables us to adapt to an ever-changing external environment based on our perceptions. Now, a system like this needs no help, just no interference!

The skeleton begins to form at around week five and six and is designed to do so until you are fully formed. Ever noticed that we all have two ears which are situated on either side of our head? Or that our eyes are situated just under our forehead in the orbital cavity and below our eyebrows? What enables this to happen? The internal wisdom of the body — the innateness of design, if you will — creates this without us consciously thinking about it. At only eleven weeks *all* the systems of the body are in working order with the muscles and nerves working together to create the first movements and the entire system fits into the size of our little finger. Ain't that grand!! Only five weeks later the baby is identifiable as a human being, with eyelids, ears, nose, mouth, fingernails, feet, and organs. All these are coordinated to enable growth and development under the watchful eye of the intelligence of life within, coupled with the governing system: the nerve system.

At around 18 weeks it is possible to clearly see the child sucking its thumb. We now know the benefit to this is the preparation for breast feeding upon birth. It also helps regulate the sacral occipital motion and the pumping of the cerebrospinal fluid around the body delivering nutrients to the nerve system and taking toxins away.

At this stage, the fetus has developed a personality of its own. It's able to grasp with its hands, swim, turn somersaults, cry, talk and punch — I am sure many mothers have felt those before! If there is no interference, the fetus shall continue to grow into a healthy human being without assistance from external sources.

At 28 weeks the fetus is considered to be viable, which means it has everything it needs to be able to live outside of its mother. Hair begins to appear, not only on the head, but on the body and eyebrows. A beautiful, cheesy-looking vernix envelops the fetus in order to protect its skin from drying. The child's sleeping patterns start to appear. The child responds to sounds in frequencies too high or too low for the adult to hear. In the next month, the eyelids open, the eye teeth become present, the mother's voice is recognized and the hand grip is strengthened.

Once the child is born, he or she will physically hear for the first time, see for the first time, experience temperature changes for the first time and breathe, using their lungs for the first time (inhaling just the right amount of oxygen), experience gravity for the first time and so forth… all this outside of its stable environment. All the organs are prepared to function at 100%. The child will do this exactly right every time, provided there is no interference. The child has within itself an endless supply of possibilities!

Although I have shared with you the journey of the unborn child in the desire to increase your awareness and respect for the intricacies of the innateness within, I want you to know within *every* living thing there is an intelligence which, if allowed to express itself without interference, will do so exactly right every time.

When Sue and Mark brought their four month old son, Ben, into the practice for care they were at a loss as to what to do and where to go professionally with their young boy. They had been told many things about Ben's "condition" and as such felt awfully confused. Upon birth Ben's parents noticed the anterior (front) to posterior (back) strain through his cranium — a twisting type of action where his left side was further forward than his right side. The left frontal, temporal and occiput were pushed forward and the right frontal, temporal and occiput were pushed backwards. Ben's parents were alarmed at the sight of his skull and sought out a pediatrician who specialized in this area so as to have a more aesthetically pleasing son to look at.

Ben's parents visited the pediatrician not long after Ben was born. Upon their visit to the pediatrician they were informed that if his cranium (skull) did not correct itself in the next few months then a helmet would be provided to the young boy to be worn constantly in order to redirect the growing of the bones so as to establish something more aesthetically appealing.

There was no mention to the parents of brain development or breast feeding advantages in situations like this. This little boy already had limitations in his neck movement and wearing a helmet at such a young age when he was unable to coordinate the head lifting movement seemed absurd to the parents.

The power of the body and the innate wisdom it carries was explained to Mark and Sue. Also explained was the daily impact the strain had on his sleep and waking patterns. Ben's limited movement from side to side was a result of in-utero constraint coupled with a challenged birth. Ben's mother was breastfeeding at the time, however was finding it challenging on the left side. One of the benefits of breast feeding, it was explained to Sue, helps the cranium to open up — especially after an adjustment. Sue was encouraged to continue with the breast feeding even in the face of the challenges. She was told it would improve.

After a series of adjustments, Ben's cranium started to balance itself. His neck movements started to become larger and overall the boy came alive. Sue and Mark took Ben back to the pediatrician's office and while she was sitting in the waiting room, she couldn't help but notice another mother sitting there with her child who was already in a helmet. Sue found she couldn't stop herself from sharing the information with the mother about her experience of regular adjustments and the impact it had made to Ben's life and their own life in such a short time. Sue sat there sharing everything with this lady until the pediatrician came out to call in the next patient. The pediatrician couldn't help but notice the changes in Ben's cranium. He was astonished at the results in such a short period of time.

B.J. Palmer says "you never know how far reaching something you may think, say or do today will affect the lives of millions tomorrow." Sue affected the life of the lady in the waiting room by sharing her story and Chiropractic affected the lives of Sue, Mark and Ben. Nature truly needs no help, just no interference.

The *Vital* Truth

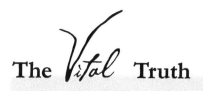

- Nature needs no help, just no interference.

- Let's not interfere with what is a natural process.

- Do you help the grass to grow? Do you help the sun to rise?

- Babies know what to do every time, all the time, in just the right sequence at just the right time in order to create limitless potential for themselves.

The *Vital* Questions

- Are you or is somebody you know pregnant? If so, find a chiropractor in your area and free the body of interference: physically, chemically and emotionally, to enable your child the best possible start to life.

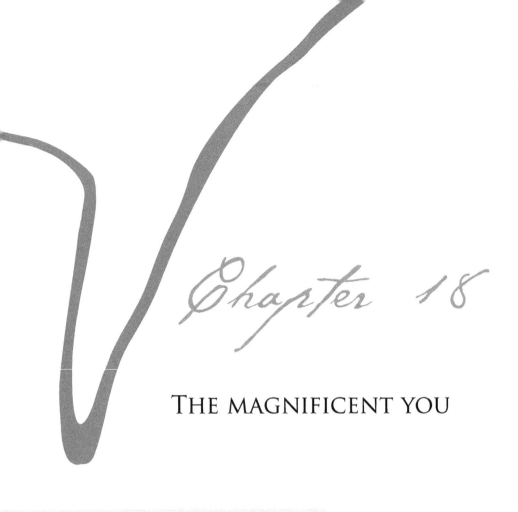

Chapter 18

THE MAGNIFICENT YOU

"Life is just a mirror, and what you see out there, you must first see inside of you"

WALLY "FAMOUS" AMOS (1936—)

It is not often that we sit and reflect on the internal workings of the body. When was the last time you thought about the heart beating or the food being digested in your stomach? In fact some people never think about it. I would like to share with you the wondrous internal workings of the body and the gift that it gives to you on a daily basis so that in turn you will have more appreciation for the life it brings to you. My intention is to also increase your awareness around the many functions taking place and how your attitude, your level of gratitude and your physical, chemical and emotional realities can have an impact on its function and the ability to keep you healthy in all areas of your life.

As you read through these remarkable facts on the body, stop to integrate them into your daily life with thanks. Always remember your body is a regenerating, self-healing, self-regulating organism which is constantly adapting to its environment and which is coordinated through the nervous system. You were born to express health to its highest level and only YOU can make it happen.

- A nerve can send up to 1000 impulses per second.

- The brain operates on the same amount of electricity as a 10 watt light bulb.

- The adult brain has 14 billion nerve cells and weighs only 3 lbs (1.5 kg).

- The brain is 85% water.

- The brain uses 25% of all the body's oxygen.

- The human brain triples in size during the first few years of childhood.

- The longest nerve is located in the leg and extends from the large toe to the spinal column.

- The pineal gland, in the centre of the skull, tells the body the time of the day and the season of the year.

- The two halves of the brain control opposite sides of the body.

- Semi circular canals in the ear have small hairs (cilia) which detect movement and direction.

- Shiny white enamel on the teeth is the hardest material in the body.

- The average person eats 3 lbs (1.5 kg) of food daily.

- Your mouth makes half a quart of saliva daily.

- Mammals have a growth factor in saliva which makes wounds heal faster.

- Saliva is 99% water.

- Enzymes in saliva digest only starchy foods.

- Dental plaque begins to develop within 6 hours of brushing.

- The heart pumps 5 liters (1.3 gallons) of blood through the body per minute and beats over 100,000 times daily.

- The human heart may beat up to 2.5 billion times in an average lifetime.

- The size of your heart is equal to that of your fist.

- The normal adult has an average heart rate of 70-72 beats per minute for men and 78-82 beats for women.

- Lungs are the only organs that float in water.

- Blood outside the body clots in about six minutes.

- A sneeze creates a force of air moving nearly 100 mph (approximately 160 km/hr).

- Humans breathe 20 times/minute over 10 million times a year and about 700 million in a lifetime.

- Only one fifth of air breathed is oxygen.

- Breathing is controlled by the muscles of the ribs and the diaphragm.

- The salivary glands pour 1.5 liters into the digestive system daily.

- The digestive system is a 30 foot (approximately 9.15m) long tube, open at both ends.

- It takes 24 hours to completely digest food.

- Surface area of the digestive system is 2,000 sq ft (approximately 186 m²).

- The stomach can stretch up to 50 times its empty size and hold about 4.5 quarts (approximately 4.25 ℓ).

- Each minute about half a million damaged lining cells are replaced in the stomach.

- Vomiting can empty not only the stomach, but the first foot (just over 30 cm) or so of the intestine.

- The small intestine averages 21 feet (6.4 m) long while the large intestine is only 5 feet (1.52 m) long.

- Water molecules in the gut move at 1500 mph (just over 2,400 km/hr).

- It takes 4-8 seconds for food to travel to the stomach.

- 94% of all the food digested is reclaimed by the small intestines.

- The color of feces comes from leftover bits of bile from the liver.

- The colon is home to 100 trillion bacteria.

- The body's bacteria could fill a soup can.

- Human feces are normally one quarter dead intestinal bacteria.

- 46% of the world population has blood type O, making it the most common type.

- There are about 62,000 miles (over 99,780 km) of blood vessels in the body – two and a half times around the world.

- Red blood cells reproduce at a rate of 8 million per second.

- The largest vein is the inferior vena cava, which drains the entire lower half of the body.

- The aorta is the largest artery and is over one inch in diameter.

- Blood supplies body tissues through capillaries, because the walls of the arteries and veins are too thick for nutrients to pass through.

- It takes one full minute for a blood cell to travel through the entire body.

- There are 200 different types of cells in the body.

- The body is made up of around 100 trillion cells.

- Only 1% of human genes differ from those of the chimpanzee.

- Fat cells are liquid at body temperature.

- There are 700 different enzymes in the body

- The body is more sensitive to pain in the afternoon.

- Shivering is the body's way of keeping warm.

- Body temperature rises by 2 degrees late in the day.

- Yawning can be the result of not breathing deeply enough.

- The "hip bone" is actually six bones joined to the sacrum to form the pelvis.

NERVE IMPULSES TRAVEL AS FAST AS 170 MILES PER HOUR (ALMOST 274 KM/HR).

- There are 230 joints in the body

- The oldest human lived to be over 120 years.

- More babies are born between 3:00 am – 4:00 am than at any other time of the day.

- Fraternal twins are the result of two eggs in the womb, while identical twins grow from a single egg.

- Fingernails grow four times faster than toenails.

- The strongest muscle of the body is the masseter muscle, located in the jaw.

- The femur is the longest bone in the body.

- You shrink half an inch (1.26 cm) during the day, due to compression of the spinal column.

- Eyes at birth are ⅔ of their mature size.

- Blue or green eyes have less pigment than brown eyes.

- One in 12 men is color blind.

- There are 6 million cones (color light-receptors) and 120 million rods (black and white light-receptors) in each eye.

- Blinking causes the eyes to be closed for an hour each day.

- Straight hair is round while curly hair is flat.

- Tiny holes on the inside of the eye carry tears into the nose.

- The average head has 100,000 hairs; each lives about 2-4 years.

- There are over 5 million hair follicles on the body — none on the lips, palms and soles of the feet.

- 50-100 scalp hairs fall out daily.

- One square inch (6.45 cm²) of skin on the back of your hand has 12,000 nerve endings.

- "Goosebumps" are the body's way of adding an extra layer of insulation.

- Fingerprints form 6-8 weeks before birth.

- 500 million dead skin cells fall off daily due to ordinary wear and tear.

- The skin is the largest organ of the body.

- There are 30 times more pain receptors than cold sensors.

- Blushing is the body cooling itself by dilating small blood vessels below the skin.

- There are 650 sweat glands in a square inch (6.45 cm²) of skin.

- Your arm span is usually equal to your height.

- There are 20 muscles located in the hand.

- All the body muscles pulling in one direction would equal 25 tons (over 22,600 kg) of force.

- The kidneys filter 180 quarts (more than 170 *l*) of blood daily.

- Fresh urine is 95% water and 5% urea.

- One quarter of all blood is filtered in the kidneys every minute.

- Urine's yellow color comes from bile, not salt.

- Bones are 1/5 of the total body weight.

- Muscles normally account for 40% of body weight.

- The average adult liver is the heaviest organ in the body at around 3lbs (1.5 kg).

- Calories burn fastest when exercise occurs within 3 hours of a meal.

- There are 26 bones in the foot.

- The last bone to mature is the collar bone.

- One in 20 people has an extra rib.

- 98% of the body is replaced every year.

- Skin cells are replaced every month.

- We receive a new stomach lining every four days.

- Bone cells are replaced every three months.

- Liver cells are replaced every six weeks.

- It takes 17 muscles to smile and 43 to frown.

- A sneeze can exceed a speed of 100 mph (almost 161 km/hr).

- There are 206 bones in the body.

- Each square inch of human skin consists of 20 feet (over 6 m) of blood vessels.

- Every square inch of the human body has an average of 32 million bacteria on it.

- We shed about 600,000 particles of skin every hour and about 1.5 pounds (almost 700 g) per year.

- The brain has approximately 100 billion nerve cells.

- Nerve impulses travel as fast as 170 miles per hour (almost 274 km/hr).

- It takes the interaction of 72 muscles to produce human speech.

- Average life of a taste bud is 10 days.

- The skull is made up of 29 bones.

- The average surface of the human intestine is 656 square feet (almost 61 m^2).

- Human skin surface is 6.5 square feet (approximately 0.6 m^2).

- 15 million blood cells die every second.

- The human body is comprised of 80% water.

- Every year approximately 98% of the atoms in your body are replaced.

- Human heart creates enough pressure to squirt blood 30 feet (over 9 m).[10]

The *Vital* Truth

- You are a self-healing, self-regulating organism that is constantly adapting to your environment.

- The power that made the body has the power to heal it.

The *Vital* Questions

- Write about a time when you were grateful for the intricacies of your body.

Chapter 19

UNLIMITED AND STORED POTENTIAL ENERGY

"There is a vitality, a life force, an energy, a quickening, that is translated into action and because there is only one of you in all time, this expression is unique. And if you block it, it will never exist through any other medium and will be lost."

MARTHA GRAHAM

Can you produce health by getting rid of disease? The answer is *no!* You need both. And yet the majority of the population appears to believe you can. Isn't the real doctor the one you're born with? The power and innate intelligence that made the body heals the body. It also enables the body to function, which is the key to health expression.

Chiropractic provides no drugs or surgery to recipients of the care. The profession is the largest non-medical health care profession in the world. It enables the whole person to reconnect with themselves and the outside world and make changes so that balance can be reached. When balance is reached the body can express health. Yet the statistics clearly indicate that most people are still making choices based on outdated models of health care.

We all have the ability to express to our highest potential. Miscommunication in the body brings with it opportunity to do and see things from another perspective. Blocks, challenges, or obstacles are merely opportunities to see a situation in another way. This miscommunication allows the innate intelligence to step back from the situation and make new inroads or neural connections into a problem or particular situation and learn how it can be dealt with. It works much the same way as when we take some time out when we have challenges at work or at home in order to see the situation differently and thus allow ourselves to make different choices around it. Remember there are always two sides to the situation.

Just as there are positive and negative charges of energy, the body operates the same way. It has the ability to "remove itself" from the challenges within its system by introducing dis-eased states. This enables the innate intelligence to take a different communication pathway, raise your awareness to a particular sign or symptom, and when the pathway is restored by realigning the neurological communication, both the innate intelligence and the educated mind can make wiser choices. There is always the potential to do things differently!

Limitless potential — or rather, opportunity — exists between the dis-ease and the neurological communication pathway when adjustments have taken place.

The ability for the body to come back into clearer communication allows for a different outcome. We have the potential to operate differently, either in a physical, chemical or emotional sphere. We have the ability to change the way we do things internally. We have the power to switch the communication on and off. We get to choose how we express health and life on a daily basis.

Many people might not want that level of responsibility as they might still have an agenda running that is keeping them addicted to a particular person, place, thing, and/or event in their lives. There is still something in it for the person in doing what they are doing — some benefit. Why would you change it if it is providing you with a benefit that nothing else at that time is providing?

When the neuronal connections are aligned it allows people to form new perceptions, which includes being grateful for the person, place, thing, or event in their lives. Different outcomes are then sought. With different outcomes as options, people attract different situations in life. The message here is you have the power to choose and change your life by listening to the innate wisdom of your body. It sends signs and symptoms to you to awaken you to the remarkable life you have led to date and the life yet to unfold in front of you.

The wiring of our neurons is remarkable. The innate intelligence of the body provides subluxations (miscommunication; less than light) — whether in the guise of physical, chemical or emotional interferences — within the system to prompt us to seek vitalistic philosophy in our life and open our eyes to what is possible. Upon receiving regular adjustments, new neural connections are formed for the ultimate gift of growth and doing life differently.

> IT SENDS SIGNS AND SYMPTOMS TO YOU TO AWAKEN YOU TO THE REMARKABLE LIFE YOU HAVE LED TO DATE AND THE LIFE YET TO UNFOLD IN FRONT OF YOU.

Have you ever been driving a car while you have been thinking about something else? When you check back in with yourself, you say, "Who was just driving the car? Did I go through any red lights?" At that point in time our subconscious was driving the car! Our subconscious mind stores all our beliefs, values and attitudes and it is from here that we form perceptions about the world and ourselves within the world. Our perceptions determine our reality and these perceptions have a large impact on our behaviors.

When looking at the behaviors we wish to change or transform, it would be wise to look at how the subconscious supports the behaviour and look at the energy charge associated with it. The body is always searching for homeostasis — the internal mechanism which is designed to provide balance. It has no judgments or preconceived ideas; it just does what it's designed to do: balance.

When we are lopsided in our search for balance, we create the miscommunication, the subluxations in a bid by the body to awaken it to do life differently, to ask different questions. In the search for the other side where the grass is supposedly greener, we are living outside of ourselves. When there is imbalance in the perceptions of our reality towards the good or the bad, the positive or negative ends, then we haven't yet awakened ourselves to the benefits we are gaining from the situation.

For some people, change is threatening. People resist change because they think of all the things in life they may lose, rather than thinking of and embracing all the things they may gain! The body and mind provide limitless potential when we are willing to embrace change and a different way of looking at our current situation.

It's interesting that when we have a situation where we don't feel entirely comfortable, if we take a break from it (the situation) — a vacation, distance ourselves, move interstate or overseas — we suddenly are able to see the situation in a whole new light. With this separation or distance, Dr Sue Brown says we see two qualities emerge: polarity and perspective. With distance a new perspective comes to bear and often we "see" the situation for the first time. A whole new light is shed on the situation.

I find the phrase a *whole new light* interesting. I feel *whole* refers to integrity, totality, completeness. When we separate ourselves from a situation and thus gain distance from it, we long to feel reconnected, whole, complete once again; to have the balance and the unity restored, if you will. The *new* is being able to see the situation through new eyes when we take that distance and listen internally to the wisdom of the body's communication, and lastly the *light* is the balance of the negative and positive within a situation, allowing us to have the light once again switched on — which ultimately leads to love. So this *whole new light* enables us to have a new perspective on a situation. This phrase enables us to make different connections with our neural wiring, which ultimately transforms our current state, allowing us to form different realities about a certain situation.

Polarity, as Dr. Brown says, is the driving force in all of nature and living things. It is responsible for the reaction of chemicals, the movement of planets, the changes in weather and the creation of life. Polarity is the essence of our relationships with the seven areas of life. When we look in each area we find opposite poles: the positive and the negative — male and female, nice and mean, war and peace, dark and light. What I find incredible about the self is that in creating changes in the way we view our life, there is constantly this desire to return to balance, to see in a whole new light.

The *Vital* Truth

- The real doctor is the one you are born with.

- The power that made the body has the power to heal the body.

- Disease is a necessary part of growth and health.

- When we live with lopsided illusions where we feel the grass is greener on the other side, we set ourselves up to live a life of imbalance.

- The innate wisdom of our body constantly wants us to be in balance, in tune, in accord with ourselves and so provides subluxations as a means of awakening us to see differently and enable a whole new light to be shed on our expression of health.

The *Vital* Questions

- Write about a situation where you clearly saw both sides of a situation: the benefits and the drawbacks.

- Why is it when we are receiving benefits from a particular situation we are happy to stay in the situation, but when there are challenges and drawbacks we want to move towards something else?

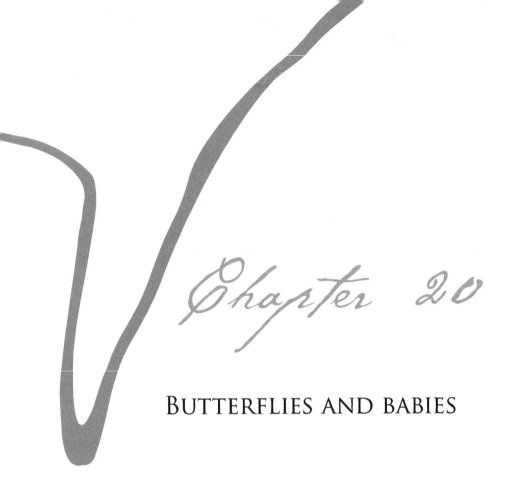

Chapter 20

BUTTERFLIES AND BABIES

"Birth in our country is one of the most profound
examples of how we have allowed the mystique of
technology to overcome practical intuition."

DR. JEANNE OHM, D.C.

It was late one afternoon when a man went outside to observe his garden. He thought he would work for awhile pulling weeds; after all the neighbour had always said to him, *"If you're not planting flowers you will be forever pulling weeds!"* He had thought about his life to date over the past few weeks and realized that he hadn't been focused on what he wanted from it. He was always helping others to reach new levels of understanding in their lives but was in a quandary over his own.

As he worked in the garden he came across a chrysalis. Watching intently, he noticed the chrysalis breaking open. He was about to witness for the first time in his life the birth of a butterfly. What he saw was a butterfly seemingly struggling with the process. The man thought, *I should help the creature.* Taking a pair of scissors, he cut through the chrysalis in the hope that it would help the butterfly to drop out of its home and into the physical world. The butterfly did just that. It dropped out easily but with compromise. The butterfly had shrunken wings and a lifeless body. He watched and watched, all the while thinking to himself that at any moment the butterfly would fly. He was waiting with anticipation for the event to happen, for its body to firm up, for the wings to spread and carry the beautiful butterfly away into the aether. The butterfly did neither. Instead it just lay there, never being able to experience what its body was designed to do.

Was nature interfered with?

What the man failed to realise was that the "struggle" the butterfly was supposedly having during the birth wasn't a struggle at all — it was the ingenious design of the innate knowing of the butterfly. The sequence of events was happening at just the right time, in just the right order and with just the right amount of pressure in order for the butterfly to reach new levels of growth, opportunity and possibility upon its birth. Here's the ingenious innate design: a butterfly, when ready to be born, pushes itself through a tiny opening at the bottom of the chrysalis and in so doing forces all the fluid from its body to the wings, which helps it to fly. What the man missed was that if you touch or pull at a butterfly's wings it is unable to fly, and without the art of flying, it perishes. Does this sound familiar to some people?

We can draw parallels with this story when understanding how humans are birthed — or rather, "delivered". Here are some questions which need to be addressed:

- Why do we allow the educated mind of others to override our own innate understanding of *our* pregnancy and birth process?

- Why do we feel safer at a hospital?

- Why do we put more faith in technology than in our innate knowing?

- Why do we attach ourselves to an arbitrary date that doesn't exist? Research tells us that only 5% of babies actually arrive on their "due date"!

- Why do we allow others to interfere with this remarkable journey, either via physical, chemical or emotional means?

Babies birth like butterflies. As they pass through the vaginal canal they create pressure changes which enable the fluid from the lungs to be expelled. This allows the baby to better adapt to life outside of the womb. Breathing takes place in just the right amounts and for the first time. Knowing what we now know about the body and its ingenious design as in the example of the butterfly, let's have a look at these questions: Does a baby need our help to develop? Does a human cell need our help to grow? The answer to these questions is *no*: nature needs no help, just no interference. So why is it that we don't allow our babies to grow and birth according to nature's plan? Elective caesarean sections rob the mother of an experience and rob the child of its rightful developmental stages. A vaginal birth triggers automatic processes which enable a cascade of vital events to take place in the physical world.

The question that demands consideration is: why do we let another person tell us what is happening inside?

If you have ever had the privilege of seeing a caterpillar in a chrysalis — its house — it truly is remarkable. A feat of greatness. You will notice that the chrysalis is built at just the right time, in just the right size and the caterpillar stays in there for just the right length of time in order for it to create its metamorphosis. There is nobody from its species trying to tell it what to do, trying to entice it to come out, or trying to predict its birth date!

"NATURE NEEDS NO HELP, JUST NO INTERFERENCE."

In the caterpillar/butterfly world, nothing exists on the outside. Everything the caterpillar needs is contained within. There is an innate intelligence, and as B.J. Palmer said, "Nature needs no help, just no interference." In the birth experience of humans, the same amazing innate intelligence exists. As we look at the beauty of Nature, we understand that humans are no different and that we only have to *look* at how Nature "does it".

The *Vital* Truth

- Nature truly needs no help, just no interference.

- Chiropractic care throughout pregnancy reduces the need for outside intervention.

The *Vital* Questions

- Do you trust in your body's ability to birth a child without outside interference?

- Are you ready to trust the innate intelligence in your own body, rather than relying on the "outside-in" approach to health?

Your notes

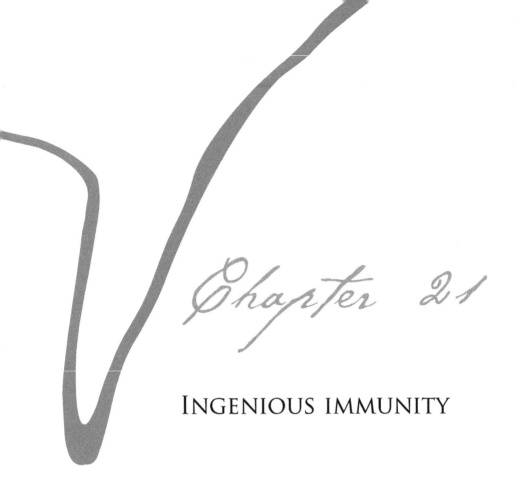

Chapter 21

INGENIOUS IMMUNITY

"Diseases are crises of purification, of toxic elimination.
Symptoms are the natural defenses of the body.
We call them diseases, but in fact they are the cure of
diseases."

HIPPOCRATES

There is much research into the efficacy of vaccinations and their effect on the body. I want to first talk about one of the most extraordinary systems in the body: the immune system, which is designed to enable growth both internally and externally. Let's first look at the internal design of the system.

The immune system is three-tiered. It has the skin and mucosa, the blood and then the lymphocytes which are divided into two types: the T and B lymphocytes. The B lymphocytes are further divided into five subcategories, each of which ultimately produces one of five different types of antibodies (immunoglobulins): A, G, M, E and D. When a toxin punctures the surface of the skin there is a whole cascade of events that take place in just the right amounts, at the right time and in the right sequence in order to take care of the entering toxin.

The skin and mucous membranes are the first line of defense, followed by the blood. Bleeding aids the body in removing the toxin from the punctured site. Notice that when we wash the blood away, more continues to flow. The body decides when it shall stop the bleeding and does so when it feels it has washed what it needs to from the body. At the same time the body instigates another series of events known as coagulation in order to heal the punctured site. How remarkable. If a toxin makes it further into the body, the blood level — the lymphocytes — form the next line of defense.

"It is a serious disease to worry over what has not occurred."

IBN GABIROL

The picture here is natural immunity. The question begging to be asked is: what happens when we bypass two of the natural immune defense levels? Answer: the body gets mighty confused! See, when a toxin — let's say, chickenpox — comes into the body via natural methods, it goes through the steps described above. The body is able to take care of it and when it does so naturally the body is able to reach new levels of internal growth and understanding. This is where I feel it is necessary to reinvent the word "toxin" in this instance. The "toxins" coming into the body via natural immunity are giving the body a gift. Notice that very young children put everything in their mouths. Contrary to common belief, this isn't just for the benefit of teeth that might be on the way but not show up for a few more months — it is actually to help them build immunity to their surrounds. How ingenious! When something drops on the ground, we don't wash it before giving it back to our children. Why, when the body is in its prime to build immunity to it surrounds? Why sterilize it? The body will do that for us, and in the process the immune system will create a "memory" of the ingested toxins so that its learning can lead to a more enhanced response the next time those toxins show up again. Save yourself some time! When we stop worrying about germs and realise that they are our friend and not our foe, we will start to see the genius inside each of our children and ourselves.

I've mentioned that the body gets mighty confused when we bypass its natural immunity. This is what happens when vaccinations are introduced into the body. They're injected or ingested into the body, bypassing some of the most important defense systems: e.g. the skin mucosa (especially the tonsils), the blood and IgA.

WHY STERILIZE IT? THE BODY WILL DO THAT FOR US, AND IN THE PROCESS THE IMMUNE SYSTEM WILL CREATE A "MEMORY" OF THE INGESTED TOXINS...

What gets triggered in vaccinations is the IgG. Now, it is important to know that under normal natural immunity IgG-producing B cells are the last — yes, *last* — to be stimulated into action. All of a sudden the IgM are the first antibody to be produced in unnatural immunity. No wonder the body is getting confused by these manufactured, unnatural introduced diseases.

What is also important to remember (and we have already discussed it in detail) are the physical, chemical and emotional (or trauma, toxin and thoughts) realities of one's body when vaccines are introduced. For example, in malnourished children vaccinations carry a high mortality rate within four weeks of the injection. This suggests that you become ill to the disease when your body is undergoing other changes, such as in this case, lack of food. A body that is functioning at 100% all the time every day for a lifetime is less likely to see its potential diminished when a "toxin" comes into its internal house. No doubt the body shall see it as an opportunity to reach new levels of understanding and reset the homeostasis mechanism to balance at a higher level.

Chiropractic care makes sure that the body is functioning to its highest potential, and as such the profession sees people who are classed as "sick" less often. Certainly children under chiropractic care are less likely to have symptomatic expression of diseased states and if they do, it has been my observation that they recover faster.

I remember hearing an immunity seminar at college on how the defenses work. It was at a time when the game of skirmish was all the rage in the USA. The example presented at this seminar began with picturing two teams: the blue team and the red team. The blue team (the external environment of the body) decides to invade the red one's territory (the internal environment). Now, the red team knows the blue ones are present because they can see blue arm bands on the sleeve of each invading member. The red team then creates a plan on how to attack the blue ones, knowing they are able to contain the blue ones because they are able to identify them. Are you getting the picture? This is just like playing skirmish — there are two teams and we're trying to attack each other to win dominance of the territory. So we can see here that the better we identify ourselves to our team, the better our team members are able to attack the right person.

Now let's paint a different picture. Let's say the red team and the blue team aren't colour coded. Wow — we can get the picture right away, can't we! Cells can't be in protection and growth at the same time. Dr. Bruce Lipton, a cell biologist at the cutting edge of research, has done experiments in this area and found this to be the case.[11] So what happens internally to the body? Well, imagine playing skirmish where nobody had any colour bands. Wouldn't we all be out there for ourselves? Of course we would. Who would we trust? My point is this: when the body goes through natural immunity, it gets to see who the players are.

What happens when a body is functioning at less than an optimal level, when a body has a compromised nerve system? It is unable to receive clear messages between the body and the brain due to interference. This interference results in the body expressing confusion in a multitude of ways when unnatural immunity is imposed. A body that is already compromised has a communication system that has interference between it and the external world. It therefore finds it exceptionally hard to adapt to the changes that are taking place.

It is wise to get your children checked for interference from a young age — ideally whilst pregnant or at least from birth, and onwards for a lifetime. Would it be wise for people, who despite all the research against the use of vaccinations still choose to do it for whatever reason, get checked? Yes, of course. A body that is communicating with itself via clear messages is more likely to gain from the experience of natural immunity and cope better if unnatural immunity is sought.

Here are some important facts from the Australian Vaccination Network (AVN) which is a wonderful organization distributing vital information to people in our communities.

- Some vaccines contain genetically engineered yeast, animal, bacterial and viral DNA;

- Some vaccines contain antibiotics such as neomycin to fight infection;

- The rubella portion of the MMR (measles, mumps and rubella) vaccine is cultured on the cell-line of an aborted human fetus;

- Live virus vaccines such as polio, measles, mumps, rubella, and chickenpox are carried in the body for up to 90 days after vaccination;

- Studies from around the world have shown that vaccines can increase the risk of allergy and auto-immunity deficiency;

- Vaccines don't guarantee protection from the disease; and

- Vaccines contain many toxic ingredients.

There is a great easy-to-read book the AVN put out to educate the public on vaccinations. The AVN point out startling realities, such as the fact that infant mortality had dropped by 80% prior to the mid-1930s, yet antibiotics and the widespread use of vaccines weren't introduced until after World War II in the 1940s. The drop in the mortality rate was actually due to socioeconomic factors such as higher standards of sanitation and nutrition.[12]

I used to take our youngest son to gymnastics. While there I met a lovely mum who had twins — a girl and a boy. We became friendly and one day she began telling me about her daughter Louise, and how since turning 18 months old she had been a recluse. Louise was not socializing or speaking. Many had called her mildly autistic, and she was attending a speech pathologist once a week. I asked more questions — what was the other twin like? What was their birth like: caesarean section or vaginal, home or hospital, drugs or no drugs? The picture began to emerge that the damage could quite possibly be due to vaccination. After a few more weeks of getting to know her I spoke to her on the phone and suggested she bring Louise in to the practice to get checked. I spoke about the nerve system and the communication pathway and the messages being unable to be read by her body to her brain and vice versa. I kept it very simple so as to not overwhelm her, and that week she brought Louise in.

After Louise's first adjustment her parents couldn't believe the changes. She was more interactive, her speech was clearer and she was asking for more! After a week, the changes were significant. The speech pathologist asked what they were doing and they mentioned the chiropractic care. The process had so impressed the speech pathologist that more parents were referred to our practice for chiropractic care.

Louise has been under care for a few years now and enjoys a life full of social activity and clear communication between her family, friends and twin brother, Charlie. The whole family is now under care and they constantly remind me of the changes that have taken place and those still occurring. They couldn't believe that nobody had recommended chiropractic to them earlier.

I share this story about Charlie and Louise for the purpose of spreading the message. As B.J. Palmer said, "You never know how far reaching something you think say or do today will affect the lives of millions tomorrow."

The *Vital* Truth

- Kids benefit immensely from regular chiropractic care from a young age.

- Allow your child's body to build immunity in a natural way, ensuring toxins reach the body's defense mechanisms in the correct order.

The *Vital* Questions

- Have you allowed fear to induce you to agree to have your child vaccinated?

- Have you taken time to properly research the premise of the vaccine argument?

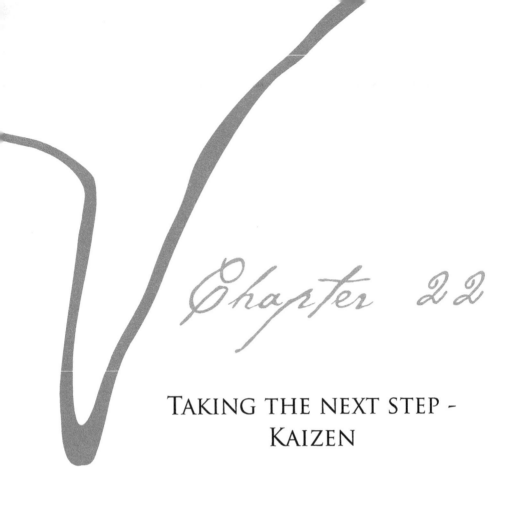

Chapter 22

TAKING THE NEXT STEP -
KAIZEN

"The journey of a thousand miles begins with the first step."

OLD PROVERB

As you read the information contained in this book, you may feel overwhelmed with the enormity of the changes you would like to implement into your life in order to create changed states in your health expression. We have covered many principles in the text along with factual accounts from myself and others I have come in contact with over the years.

The book is based on three basic principles:

1.   Health exists on a continuum;

2.   The power that made the body heals the body;

3.   Nature needs no help, just no interference.

When acknowledged and integrated into our lives, these principles have a great impact on the manifestation of health and vitality, and the choices we make on a daily basis influence the expression of them. We are all self-healing, self-regulating organisms who are constantly adapting to our environment.

"The Vital Questions" were designed to trigger different ways of thinking, to encourage different questions to be asked. If done in accordance with each chapter, great insights can be made and the changes are rapid. Internal channels become unlocked and new information floods the body in its quest to seek new understanding in our life.

Rather than feeling overwhelmed at the enormity of the information provided, take small steps in the changes you make. Remember the book can be picked up and put down in order to absorb new ideas gradually. It is all about taking at least a step in the direction of looking at health and its expression in a different way. Some readers will, no doubt, take huge leaps and bounds in their quest for greater balance and expression of health in all seven areas of their life, and others will require a method to follow.

One method I suggest is based on Kaizen[13]. Originating in Japan, *Kaizen* is interpreted as *continuous improvement* and is seen as a way-of-life philosophy. Proponents of this method accept that change is imminent in our life and every aspect of it deserves to be continually improved. Kaizen espouses simple, specific, gradual and continuous change. As the old proverb says "The journey of a thousand miles begins with the first step."

In acknowledging that small, gradual and continual steps are beneficial in sustaining change, we can move forward to look at how to integrate the changes we wish to see in our lives.

If you go back to Diagram 5F(A) and (B) where we plotted the seven areas of life on the wheel, you will be able to see where the support and challenges are occurring at present. Consider where in the seven areas of life you would like to have greater balance. Take the least challenging area to begin implementing different ways of doing your life. For example, if the familial area was low on the wheel of life, ask yourself, "What would be three *simple* steps to make changes in my family interactions?" Remember, Kaizen says to keep it simple, specific, gradual and continuous. It might be as simple as telling your partner you love them.

We can choose to embrace this new understanding of health, where it comes from, how to get it, and how to keep it — or we can choose to continue as we have always done. Einstein said "Insanity is doing the same thing over and over again and expecting different results."

Do you want to revolve or evolve?

Are you ready to implement the change you have been looking for?

Are you ready to receive?

Your notes

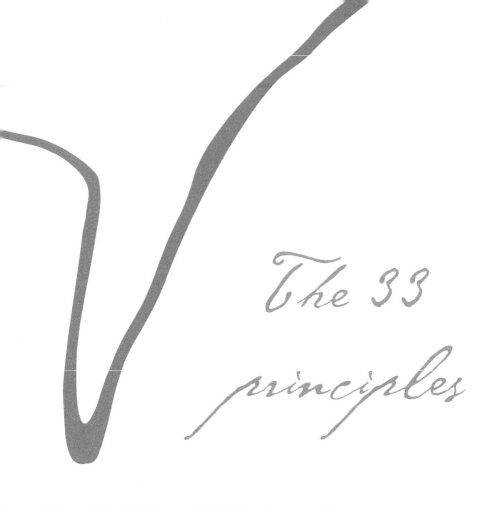

The 33 principles

"Get the big idea, all else follows."

B.J. PALMER

1. THE MAJOR PREMISE:

A Universal Intelligence is in all matter and continually gives to it all its properties and actions, thus maintaining it in existence.

2. THE CHIROPRACTIC MEANING OF LIFE:

The Expression of this intelligence through matter is the Chiropractic meaning of life.

3. THE UNION OF INTELLIGENCE AND MATTER:

Life is necessarily the union of intelligence and matter.

4. THE TRIUNE OF LIFE:

Life is a tri-unity, having three necessary united factors: Intelligence, Force and Matter.

5. THE PERFECTION OF THE TRIUNE:

In order to have 100% Life, there must be 100% Intelligence, 100% Force, 100% Matter.

6. THE PRINCIPLE OF TIME:

There is no process that does not require time.

7.   THE AMOUNT OF INTELLIGENCE IN MATTER:

The amount of intelligence for any given amount of matter is 100%, and is always proportional to its requirements.

8.   THE FUNCTION OF INTELLIGENCE:

The function of intelligence is to create force.

9.   THE AMOUNT OF FORCE CREATED BY INTELLIGENCE:

The amount of force created by intelligence is always 100%.

10.   THE FUNCTION OF FORCE:

The function of force is to unite intelligence and matter.

11.   THE CHARACTER OF UNIVERSAL FORCES:

The forces of Universal Intelligence are manifested by physical laws; are unswerving and unadapted, and have no solicitude for the structures in which they work.

12.   INTERFERENCE WITH TRANSMISSION OF UNIVERSAL FORCES:

There can be interference with transmission of universal forces.

13. THE FUNCTION OF MATTER:

The function of matter is to express force.

14. UNIVERSAL LIFE:

Force is manifested by motion in matter; all matter has motion, therefore there is universal life in all matter.

15. NO MOTION WITHOUT THE EFFORT OF FORCE:

Matter can have no motion without the application of force by intelligence.

16. INTELLIGENCE IN BOTH ORGANIC AND INORGANIC MATTER:

Universal Intelligence gives force to both organic and inorganic matter.

17. CAUSE AND EFFECT:

Every effect has a cause and every cause has effects.

18. EVIDENCE OF LIFE:

The signs of life are evidence of the intelligence of life.

19. ORGANIC MATTER:

The material of the body of a "living thing" is organized matter.

20. INNATE INTELLIGENCE:

A "living thing" has an inborn intelligence within its body, called Innate Intelligence.

21. THE MISSION OF INNATE INTELLIGENCE:

The mission of Innate Intelligence is to maintain the material of the body of a "living thing" in active organization.

22. THE AMOUNT OF INNATE INTELLIGENCE:

There is 100% of Innate Intelligence in every "living thing" the requisite amount, proportional to its organization.

23. THE FUNCTION OF INNATE INTELLIGENCE:

The function of Innate Intelligence is to adapt universal forces and matter for use in the body, so that all parts of the body will have co-coordinated action for mutual benefit.

24. THE LIMITS OF ADAPTATION:

Innate Intelligence adapts forces and matter for the body as long as it can do so without breaking a universal law, or Innate Intelligence is limited by the limitations of matter.

25. THE CHARACTER OF INNATE FORCES:

The forces of Innate Intelligence never injure or destroy the structures in which they work.

26. COMPARISON OF UNIVERSAL AND INNATE FORCES:

In order to carry on the universal cycle of life, Universal forces are destructive, and Innate forces constructive, as regards structural matter.

27. THE NORMALITY OF INNATE INTELLIGENCE:

Innate Intelligence is always normal and its function is always normal.

28. THE CONDUCTORS OF INNATE FORCES:

The forces of Innate Intelligence operate through or over the nervous system in animal bodies.

29. INTERFERENCE WITH TRANSMISSION OF INNATE FORCES:

There can be interference with the transmission of innate forces.

30. THE CAUSES OF DIS-EASE:

Interference with the transmission of innate forces causes incorporation of dis-ease.

31. SUBLUXATIONS:

Interference with transmission in the body is always directly or indirectly due to subluxations in the spinal column.

32. THE PRINCIPLE OF COORDINATION:

Coordination is the principal of harmonious action of all the parts of an organism, in fulfilling their offices and purposes.

33. THE LAW OF DEMAND AND SUPPLY:

The Law of Demand and Supply is existent in the body in its ideal state; wherein the "clearing house" is the brain, Innate the virtuous "banker," brain cells "clerks," and nerve cells "messengers."

About the Author

There are only a few times in someone's life where an inspirational person comes along with a different and profound message to share — a person who challenges conventional understanding and breaks out of existing paradigms of thought.

Dr. Sarah Farrant is a woman whose experience, knowledge and philosophy are clearly ahead of their time.

As an international speaker she enables people to have their minds opened, moving them to new and exciting opportunities and possibilities. When she speaks, people listen. Her revolutionary way of looking at health and vitality are reshaping how people see themselves and their health not only at an individual level but at family, community, city, state, national and global levels.

For more information about Dr. Sarah Farrant go to www.drsarahfarrant.com or contact info@drsarahfarrant.com

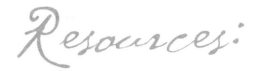

UNIQUE LEADERSHIP

DR. SARAH FARRANT, D.C. : www.drsarahfarrant.com

Dr. Farrant is a pioneer in the way health is taught across the world. An innovative thinker and educator, she is reshaping how people define health, where it comes from, how to get it and how to keep it. Dr. Farrant holds a degree in Physical Education, a Graduate Diploma in Psychology, a Degree in General Science and a Doctor of Chiropractic, all of which form a foundation for the knowledge and experience she shares with audiences. Dr. Farrant's ideas are innovative and her interpretation is unique.

DR. SUE BROWN, D.C. : www.bgiseminars.com

Dr. Brown is the owner of Essence Quality of Life Center, located in the western suburbs of Chicago. Her experience both in practice and teaching, as well as her studies and theories of force dynamics and seismic events as they relate to the formation of subluxations, and the sacred geometry of the body have provided her with both a unique perspective and new approaches to the dynamics of Chiropractic.

DR. ARNO BRUNIER, D.C. : www.masterpiece-seminars.com
& www.cafeoflife.com

Dr. Brunier has inspired audiences throughout the world with his heart, experience, insight and simplicity. Through Arno's various lectures, seminars and training camps, he shares his expertise and offers his unique experience as a husband, parent, teacher, mentor and chiropractor. Arno Brunier, D.C. has a rare view of Chiropractic's "Big Idea" as well as an amazing ability to reach into your mind, heart and soul.

DR. JOHN DEMARTINI, D.C. : www.drdemartini.com

Founder of the Concourse School of Wisdom, Dr Demartini teaches personal and professional development. His words of wisdom inspire minds, open hearts and motivate people to action.

DR. BRUCE LIPTON, PH.D. : www.brucelipton.com

Dr. Bruce Lipton has accomplished groundbreaking work in the field of New Biology. He shows how our perceptions and beliefs, be them good or bad, are able to affect our genetic coding and expression.

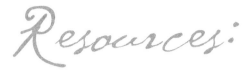

ORGANIZATIONS

LIFE CHIROPRACTIC COLLEGE ATLANTA, USA:
www.life.edu

NEW ZEALAND CHIROPRACTIC COLLEGE, AUCKLAND, NZ:
www.nzchiro.co.nz

PALMER COLLEGE OF CHIROPRACTIC, IOWA, USA:
www.palmer.edu

> In my opinion these three schools are the leading schools in the profession. All three represent the art, science and philosophy of the chiropractic profession.

TRUE FOOD GUIDE: http://sites.greenpeace.org.au/truefood/index2.html

> This website has information to stay true to the foods we choose to consume. It has information about which companies use genetically engineered products in the manufacturing process.

AUSTRALIAN VACCINATION NETWORK: www.avn.org.au

This website is dedicated to individuals who want to make informed choices about their own, their community's and their children's health. It is supportive in providing information in a readable way to consumers. The network has a magazine called "Informed Voice" which enables people to digest the material in an easy to read format. This website also houses a reading section to help increase community awareness on certain sensitive subjects.

INTERNATIONAL CHIROPRACTIC PEDIATRIC ASSOCIATION (ICPA): www.icpa4kids.com

International Chiropractic Pediatric Association (ICPA) is the oldest and largest non-profit organization of its kind. Their membership is composed of over two thousand chiropractic doctors and students around the world. These members share a common interest in the advancement of quality chiropractic care for children. The ICPA's mission is to provide education and training to members as well as supporting research on chiropractic care in pregnancy and throughout childhood.

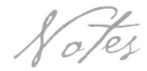

(ENDNOTES)

1. *Divided Legacy: A History of the Schism of Medical Thought*, Volume IV. Copyright © 1994 Harris Livermore Coulter. Published by North Atlantic Books, PO Box 12327, Berkeley, California 94701-9998. Also published by Center for Empirical Medicine, 4221 45th Street NW, Washington, DC 20016.

2. Ron Law, Executive Director of the National Nutritional Foods Association (NNFA), in New Zealand and member of the New Zealand Ministry of Health Working Group advising on medical error, listed these findings in an emailed response to the British Medical Journal. (November 11, 2000;321:1178A)

3. www.nhmrc.gov.au/

4. www.masaru-emoto.net/english

5. Quoted in L. I. Ponomarev, *The Quantum Dice*

6. Palmer, D.D. *The Chiropractor's Adjuster: Text-Book of the Science, Art and Philosophy of Chiropractic for Students and Practitioners* Portland Printing House Company. Portland, OR. 1910., p.552

7. *Dorland's Pocket Medical Dictionary, 24th Edition* © 1989 W.B Saunders Company

8. *The Biology of Belief: Unleashing the power of Consciousness, Matter and Miracles* Copyright © 2005, Bruce Lipton. Published by Mountain of Love/ Elite Books, Santa Rosa, CA 95404

9. From D.D. Palmer, *The Chiropractor,* 1914

10. *The Incredible Anatomical Body Maze Poster,* Copyright: 1992 Anatomical Chart Company, Skokie, Illinois, USA

11. For further information on Dr. Bruce Lipton's work, visit www.brucelipton.com

12. *Vaccination — Investigate before you vaccinate: A guide for parents.* Researched and written by Kathy Scarborough B.Sc., Grad. Dip. Ed. © 1988. Contact Vaccination Information South Australia, PO Box 643, Magill S.A., 5072.

13. http://www.12manage.com/methods_kaizen.html

Contact Details

FOR MORE INFORMATION ABOUT DR. SARAH FARRANT GO TO

www.drsarahfarrant.com

or contact

info@drsarahfarrant.com